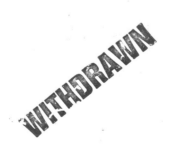

To Kay,
James, Owen and Bethan

Introduction to Clinical Immunology

Mansel Haeney, MSc, MB, BCh, MRCP, MRCPath
Consultant Immunologist, Clinical Sciences Building, Hope Hospital, Salford

Butterworths
London   Boston   Durban   Singapore   Sydney
Toronto   Wellington

Update Publications
London

First published, 1985

© Update, 1985

British Library Cataloguing in Publication Data

Haeney, Mansel
  An introduction to clinical immunology.
  1: Immunology
  I. Title
  616.07'9 QR181

  ISBN 0-407-00362-2

Library of Congress Cataloging in Publication Data

Haeney, Mansel.
  An introduction to clinical immunology.
  Rev. and expanded articles originally
  published in Hospital update.
  Includes index.
  1. Immunologic diseases. 2. Immunopathology.
  I. Title. II. Hospital update. [DNLM: 1. Autoimmune
  Diseases. 2. Immunity. 3. Immunologic Deficiency
  Syndromes. QW 504 H135i]
  RC582.H34 1984 616.07'9 84-9564

  ISBN 0-407-00362-2

Photoset by Butterworths Litho Preparation Department
Printed by Cambus Litho Ltd, Scotland
Bound by Anchor Brendon, Tiptree, Essex

Preface

Clinical immunology is the application of immunological principles to achieving a better understanding of the mechanisms of human diseases, more appropriate laboratory investigations and so more rational and effective therapy.

Immunologically mediated diseases permeate all the traditional clinical specialities but the fact that clinical immunology has so far achieved only a limited impact on patient management underlines the progress yet to be made in fully appreciating the complexities of the human immune system. Nevertheless, at moments of optimism, clinical immunologists believe they are on the verge of a new era – a time when immunology will make major contributions to health care.

Immunology is a flourishing discipline. In recent years, basic immunologists have generated a formidable literature of scientific observations, sometimes so rapidly that even workers in this field have difficulty in keeping pace with developments. The situation is even more perplexing for doctors who had minimal immunology teaching during their undergraduate or postgraduate years: many have little idea where to begin in familiarizing themselves with the scope of clinical immunology.

This book is based on series of articles commissioned by *Hospital Update*. Each chapter has been revised and three new chapters added. This is not a textbook: it is neither comprehensive nor balanced, and is thus not intended to supplant those existing, larger volumes of clinical immunology which use an organ-based approach. Instead, I have tried to provide an introduction to clinical immunology for junior doctors in training, but I hope it will also be of value to more senior clinical investigators in all disciplines who find themselves reluctantly obliged to acquire the rudiments of immunology in order to interpret important new developments in their own fields.

M. Haeney

Acknowledgements

It is a pleasure to acknowledge my debt to the Staff of the Department of Immunology, University of Birmingham and the Regional Immunology Laboratory, East Birmingham Hospital, who first stimulated and fed my interest in clinical immunology. I also want to thank Mrs Anne Patterson of Update and Mr Charles Fry of Butterworths for their unfailing help and advice. The Staff of the Illustration Department at Update deserve a special mention for their ability to convert my hesitant drawings into superb colour illustrations. I would like to express my appreciation to Mrs Eileen Walker, who skilfully interpreted so many corrected typescripts.

Finally, to my wife and children I can only express my deepest appreciation for their patience because, without their loving support and encouragement, this book would never have been possible.

Contents

1 Immunoglobulins and disease   1

2 Monoclonal immunoglobulins   9

3 IgE and atopic disease   19

4 Complement and disease   35

5 Immune complexes and disease   48

6 Antibody deficiency   64

7 Defects of cell-mediated immunity   84

8 Disorders of neutrophil function   99

9 An overview of autoimmune disease   109

Index   127

1   Immunoglobulins and disease

Basic immunoglobulin structure

All antibodies belong to the group of proteins called immunoglobulins. Every immunoglobulin molecule has a fundamentally similar structure made up of two identical 'heavy' polypeptide chains attached to a pair of identical 'light' chains (*Figure 1.1*). Analysis of different myeloma light chains shows that the amino acid sequences of the N-terminal halves of these chains vary greatly: in contrast, the C-terminal halves are almost identical. These two segments are called the variable (V_L) and constant (C_I) regions of the light chain. Heavy chain amino acid sequences show a similar pattern: a variable region (V_H) occupies the N-terminal quarter of the chain and is of similar length to the V_L region (110 amino acids), but the heavy chain constant region (C_H) is about three times longer.

An antibody molecule has two characteristic functions: (1) antigen recognition and (2) antigen elimination through participation in effector mechanisms. These functions are performed by different regions of the molecule. The proteolytic enzyme papain will split an immunoglobulin into three parts of similar size (*Figure 1.2*). Two of the fragments are identical, each containing one site capable of specific combination with antigen. These antigen-binding fragments (Fab) consist of the entire light chain, the V_H region and part of the C_H region. The third fragment is composed of the C-terminal halves of the heavy chains but does not combine with antigen. This crystallizable fragment (Fc) mediates the effector functions of an immunoglobulin which has combined with specific antigen via its Fab regions.

Immunoglobulin classes

Although all immunoglobulins have a similar basic subunit structure, five classes of heavy chain can be identified from structural differences in their C_H regions: these are called α,

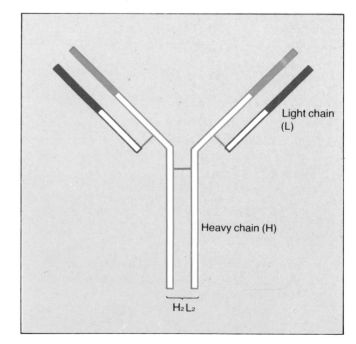

Figure 1.1 *Basic four-chain (H_2L_2) structure of immunoglobulins. The molecule is usually represented in the form of a Y with the amino (N-) termini of the four chains at the top and the carboxyl (C-) termini of the heavy chains at the bottom*

γ, δ, ε and μ and define the corresponding immunoglobulin classes IgA, IgG, IgD, IgE and IgM (*Table 1.1*). Some classes can be divided further into subclasses; for example, IgG is divisible into IgG_1, IgG_2, IgG_3 and IgG_4 subclasses. There are also two major types of light chain, designated kappa and lambda, associated with the heavy chains of all

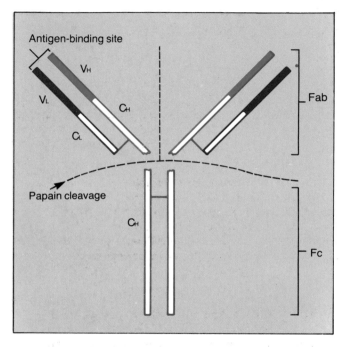

Figure 1.2 *Immunoglobulin fragments produced by papain digestion. The antigen-binding site is contained within the Fab region and formed by the variable regions of one heavy and one light chain. Each monomeric immunoglobulin possesses two antigen-binding sites per molecule*

immunoglobulins. In other words, the class of an immunoglobulin molecule depends on the constituent heavy chain and is independent of the light chain type. A single immunoglobulin molecule has identical light and identical heavy chains.

Immunoglobulin classes also differ in the number of basic H_2L_2 subunits in the molecule (*Table 1.1*). IgG, IgD and IgE are each made up of one subunit. Most of the IgA in normal serum is composed of a single subunit (monomeric IgA),

but the rest, and much of the IgA in secretions, consists of two subunits linked to an extra polypeptide chain (secretory component) to form secretory IgA. Secretory component is a product of intestinal epithelial cells and protects the molecule from proteolytic digestion in the intestinal lumen. Serum IgM is a pentamer of five subunits and therefore has 10 antigen-binding sites. Dimers and pentamers are stabilized by a further polypeptide (J chain) synthesized by plasma cells.

Immunoglobulin structure versus function

The B lymphocyte response to a single antigen may include specific antibody molecules of all five immunoglobulin classes. Antibodies of different classes may show identical antigen-binding specificities and thus presumably may possess identical variable ($V_H + V_L$) regions; however, the C_H regions mediate different secondary effector functions (*Table 1.2*).

Complement activation

The classical pathway of complement activation is initiated by the binding of the C1q subcomponent to the IgM or IgG component of an antigen–antibody complex. An alternative pathway of complement activation, triggered by cell wall endotoxins in conjunction with a series of serum factors, can bypass the need for antibody, C1, C4 or C2 complement components and allow direct cleavage of C3. IgM and IgG can also activate this alternative pathway under certain circumstances but it is unclear whether other immunoglobulin classes do so *in vivo* (see Chapter 4).

Binding to cells

Some immunoglobulins are bound to cell surfaces. Phagocytic cells (monocytes, macrophages and polymorphs) have receptors which recognize sites in the constant regions of IgG molecules. Foreign particles coated with IgG antibodies are bound by these receptors, so triggering rapid phagocytosis.

Table 1.1 Immunoglobulin classes

	IgG	IgA	IgM	IgD	IgE
Heavy chain class	γ	α	μ	δ	ϵ
Heavy chain subclasses	$\gamma_1\gamma_2\gamma_3\gamma_4$	$\alpha_1\alpha_2$	$\mu_1\mu_2$	–	–
Light chain type	$\varkappa$ or λ	$\varkappa$ or λ	$\varkappa$ or λ	$\varkappa$ or λ	$\varkappa$ or λ
Molecular formulae	$\gamma_2\varkappa_2$ $\gamma_2\lambda_2$	$\alpha_2\varkappa_2$ $\alpha_2\lambda_2$ $(\alpha_2\varkappa_2)_2.SC.J.$ $(\alpha_2\lambda_2)_2.SC.J.$	$(\mu_2\varkappa_2)_5.J.$ $(\mu_2\lambda_2)_5.J.$	$\delta_2\varkappa_2$ $\delta_2\lambda_2$	$\epsilon_2\varkappa_2$ $\epsilon_2\lambda_2$
Percentage of total serum immunoglobulins	73	20	6	<1	<0.01
Half-life (days)	23	6	5	3	2

Some cells can interact with IgG-coated foreign cells to produce contact lysis rather than phagocytosis: this process is called antibody-dependent cell-mediated cytotoxicity (ADCC) and the effector cells are termed killer (K) cells. IgE antibodies are bound to tissue-fixed mast cells via sites in their Fc regions. If an antigen combines with two adjacent IgE molecules, the resulting configurational change is believed to expose a further Fc site that initiates mast cell degranulation and the release of vasoactive amines (see Chapter 3).

Table 1.2 Biological properties of the Fc region of immunoglobulin molecules

	IgG*	IgA	IgM	IgD	IgE
Complement fixation:					
Classical pathway	+	–	+++	–	–
Alternative pathway	+	(+?)	+	–	(+?)
Binding to mononuclear cells	+	–	–	–	–
Binding to mast cells/basophils	–	–	–	–	+
Placental transfer	+	–	–	–	–
Control of catabolic rate	+	+	+	+	+

*Some subclasses only

Placental transfer

The placental transfer of immunoglobulins provides the newborn infant with an adequate repertoire of antibody specificities. In humans, only IgG antibodies cross the placenta: this is a property of the Fc region which interacts with receptors on placental syncytiotrophoblast. The Fab fragment, although one-third the size of the whole molecule, is not transferred.

Primary and secondary antibody responses

When a normal individual is first exposed to a foreign antigen, there is a lag phase lasting up to 10–12 days before antibodies appear in serum or body fluids (*Figure 1.3*). This primary antibody response is typically IgM. The time needed to reach maximal antibody levels and the duration of the peak titre varies with the nature of the antigen and the method of immunization. Subsequent encounter with the same antigen usually evokes an enhanced secondary (or memory) response characterized by:
(1) a lower threshold dose of antigen;
(2) a shorter lag phase;
(3) higher titres of antibody;
(4) persistence of antibody synthesis;
(5) predominant synthesis of IgG antibodies.

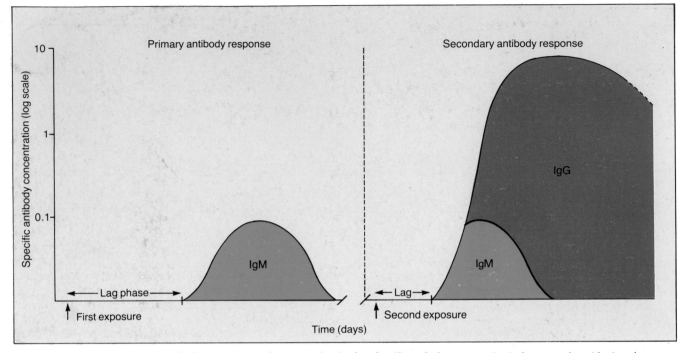

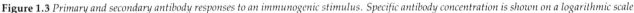

Figure 1.3 *Primary and secondary antibody responses to an immunogenic stimulus. Specific antibody concentration is shown on a logarithmic scale*

Immune response genes

In inbred experimental animals, specific responsiveness to some antigens is known to be under the control of autosomal dominant genes inherited in strict mendelian fashion and linked to the major histocompatibility complex (MHC). Immune response (Ir) genes usually have been defined by measuring the amount of antibody synthesized in response to a restricted antigenic challenge. Mice with different Ir alleles can be grouped into high or low responder strains but mice that are high responders to some antigens may be low responders to others. Ir genes do not therefore control general immune responsiveness but show antigen specificity. Genetic control of the immune response has now been demonstrated in mice, rats, guinea pigs, chickens and monkeys. The existence of Ir genes in man could explain the variable nature of the response to a

given vaccine in the population and those instances of diseases showing strong association with a particular histocompatibility type (for example, ankylosing spondylitis and HLA-B27).

Immunoglobulin levels and age

Serum immunoglobulin levels are fairly constant in healthy adults but the development of adult levels from birth shows a characteristic trend for each immunoglobulin (*Figure 1.4*). Only IgG can cross the placenta; although transfer of maternal IgG to the fetus begins as early as the thirteenth week of pregnancy, maximum transfer takes place in the last trimester. Premature infants therefore have low IgG levels and show marked susceptibility to infection. At birth, the serum IgG is wholly maternal in origin: catabolism of

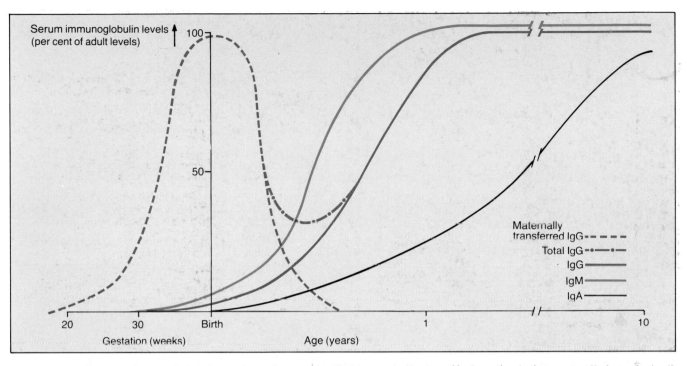

Figure 1.4 *Serum immunoglobulin levels and age. Maternally transmitted IgG has mostly disappeared by 6 months. As the neonate actively synthesizes IgG the level slowly rises, but a physiological trough of serum IgG is characteristically seen between 3 and 6 months*

this transferred IgG produces a fall in serum levels which is only partly compensated by endogenous IgG synthesis stimulated by exposure to environmental antigens. Although adult levels are reached by the age of 2 years the period between 3 and 6 months is a phase of relative antibody deficiency ('physiological trough').

Placental transfer of IgM is negligible, but fetal production of specific IgM rises to very high levels in intrauterine infection and may be of diagnostic significance. In normal infants, the serum IgM level rises rapidly in the first few months of life, reaching the adult range at between 6 months and 1 year.

IgA is not detectable in cord blood. Its appearance in serum and secretions is more gradual than IgG or IgM and adult levels are not achieved until adolescence.

IgE does not cross the placenta. Serum levels follow a similar course to IgA, adult levels being reached at between 7 and 9 years.

Abnormalities of immunoglobulins

Concept of polyclonality and monoclonality

Each immunoglobulin is the product of a single family or clone of plasma cells. Many different clones are involved in the specific antibody response but only one clone will synthesize and secrete a particular V_H and V_L region.

The malignant proliferation of a clone of plasma cells results in the increased production of immunoglobulin molecules of identical class, subclass, V_H and V_L regions. Such monoclonal immunoglobulins have a unique amino

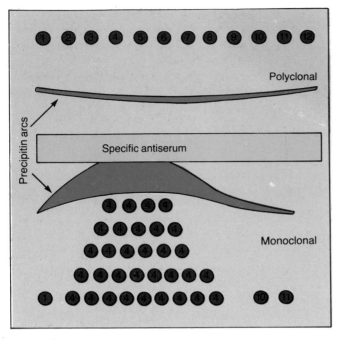

Figure 1.5 *Schematic representation of monoclonal immunoglobulin detection. A normal serum immunoglobulin class is polyclonal, that is, composed of many different antibody specificities, here represented by immunoglobulins ① to ⑫ which are synthesized by different clones of cells. The malignant proliferation of a single clone of cells produces antibody of a single specificity (for example ④) with a distinct electrophoretic mobility. The monoclonal protein is detected by its characteristic precipitin arc on immunoelectrophoresis using an antiserum specific for different heavy and light chains*

acid sequence and a finite electrophoretic mobility (*Figure 1.5*).

Polyclonal hyperimmunoglobulinaemia

Significance of raised serum immunoglobulin levels

Although statistically significant differences in serum immunoglobulin levels between healthy controls and groups of patients with various conditions can be demonstrated, immunoglobulin estimations are rarely diagnostic in an individual case. However, considered in conjunction with other laboratory findings, they may help to distinguish between diseases with otherwise similar clinical features.

Immunoglobulin patterns in disease

Some typical patterns of polyclonal increase in immunoglobulins found in disease are shown in *Table 1.3*.

Infection

Acute viral infections such as infectious mononucleosis and hepatitis A are characteristically accompanied by an IgM primary response to the antigenic challenge. Chronic

Table 1.3 Raised serum immunoglobulins: common patterns in disease

Immunoglobulin class response			Typical examples
IgG	IgA	IgM	
		√	Acute viral infection 　Hepatitis A 　Infectious mononucleosis Primary biliary cirrhosis
	√		Acute respiratory or intestinal infection Coeliac disease
√			Autoimmune disease 　SLE 　Chronic active hepatitis 　Hashimoto's thyroiditis
√	√		Chronic respiratory disease 　Tuberculosis 　Extrinsic allergic alveolitis 　Cystic fibrosis Portal cirrhosis Leprosy
√	√		Chronic bacterial infection 　Subacute bacterial endocarditis 　Subphrenic abscess 　Osteomyelitis 　Empyema Neutrophil dysfunction

respiratory or gastrointestinal infections, particularly of mycobacterial or fungal origin, stimulate a marked increase in both IgG and IgA. Long-standing bacterial infections, for example subacute bacterial endocarditis or a subphrenic abscess, are associated with significant elevations of all immunoglobulin classes.

Hepatic and gastrointestinal disease

Serum immunoglobulin levels can be of value in liver disease (*Table 1.3*), particularly when considered with the autoantibody pattern. In contrast, patients with inflammatory bowel disease rarely show significant alterations in immunoglobulin levels, although a minor elevation of IgA sometimes occurs. A persistently raised IgA is frequently a feature of gluten-sensitive enteropathy and occasionally of cow's-milk-protein intolerance. Dietary restriction of the offending antigen is usually accompanied by a fall in serum IgA, but some patients with intestinal lymphoma complicating coeliac disease show rising IgA levels despite strict dietary control.

Rheumatic diseases

Serum immunoglobulin levels are of little diagnostic value in rheumatoid arthritis or the seronegative arthritides. Total immunoglobulin and IgG levels may be moderately raised in seropositive rheumatoid disease. Sometimes, elevation of IgA is found in both seropositive and seronegative subjects but IgM levels are usually normal, irrespective of rheumatoid factor activity. In a few patients rheumatoid arthritis is associated with selective IgA deficiency. In active systemic lupus erythematosus (SLE), very high IgG levels may be produced.

Immunoglobulin levels in cerebrospinal fluid

Significant changes in serum immunoglobulin levels seldom occur in diseases of the nervous system, with the exception of SLE (see above) or dystrophia myotonica where a low IgG level results from an increased catabolic rate. In contrast, cerebrospinal fluid (CSF) IgG estimation may be of considerable diagnostic value (*Table 1.4*). In most

inflammatory diseases of the central nervous system, the integrity of the blood–brain barrier is compromised; serum 'leaks' into CSF and both CSF IgG and albumin concentrations show a proportionate increase. In demyelinating disease (*Table 1.5*), IgG appears to be locally synthesized; IgG-secreting plasma cells can be demonstrated and CSF IgG shows a restricted electrophoretic mobility. The use of a CSF IgG/albumin index controls for fluctuations in serum

Table 1.4 Changes in CSF protein concentrations (N = normal; ↑ = raised)

	Demyelinating disease	Inflammatory disease
CSF IgG	↑	↑
CSF total protein	N	↑
CSF albumin	N	↑
$\dfrac{\text{CSF IgG}}{\text{CSF total protein}}$ %	↑	N
CSF IgG/albumin index	↑	N

levels and for any increase in permeability of the blood–brain barrier. The index provides an indirect measure of local IgG synthesis and is derived as follows:

$$\text{IgG/albumin index} = \frac{\text{CSF/serum IgG ratio}}{\text{CSF/serum albumin ratio}}$$

Since both IgG and albumin ratios show a positive correlation with age, the index is age independent.

The amount of immunoglobulin synthesized intrathecally can be calculated also from an empirically derived formula (Tourtellotte's formula). This immunoglobulin is derived from so relatively few clones of plasma cells that it shows restricted heterogeneity and appears as discrete bands on CSF electrophoresis, a picture termed 'oligoclonal banding'. The detection of oligoclonal CSF IgG bands is generally recognized to be the most discriminating test of local IgG synthesis with the central nervous system: it picks up over 90% of cases of multiple sclerosis. However, this

Table 1.5 Diseases showing increased IgG synthesis in CSF

Multiple sclerosis

Other conditions
    Subacute sclerosing panencephalitis
    Viral meningoencephalitis
    Mumps meningitis
    Bacterial meningitis and brain abscess
    Neurosyphilis
    Congenital infections
    Polyneuritis

technique is not widely available but in such circumstances the IgG/albumin index will still give a correct detection rate of about 80%.

IgD and disease

No clear evidence exists of a biological role for circulating IgD: there is an apparent absence of any major antibody activity or known effector function mediated by this class of immunoglobulin. The clinical significance of serum IgD levels in disease is therefore uncertain. Many healthy people have barely detectable levels and there is little diagnostic information to be obtained from measurement of serum IgD concentration other than in cases of IgD myeloma.

IgE and disease

The role of IgE in disease is discussed more fully in Chapter 3.

Further reading

HOBBS, J. R. (1970) Immune globulins in some diseases. *British Journal of Hospital Medicine*, **3**, 669–680
LEIBOWITZ, S. and HUGHES, R. A. C. (1983) *Immunology of the Nervous System*. Arnold, London
THOMPSON, R. A. (1979) *The Practice of Clinical Immunology*, 2nd edn. Arnold, London
TURNER, M. W. (1983) The immunoglobulins. In *Immunology in Medicine*, 2nd edn (E. J. Holborow and W. G. Reeves, eds). Academic Press, London

2 Monoclonal immunoglobulins

A proliferating clone of B lymphocytes or plasma cells will synthesize immunoglobulin molecules or fragments with a common and unique protein structure. Such homogeneous monoclonal tumour cell products (*Table 2.1*) are termed paraproteins or 'M' components.

Clinical significance of monoclonal proteins

The incidence of serum paraproteins increases with age (*Table 2.2*). Three-quarters of all hospital patients with paraproteins have, or will develop, malignant tumours of B lymphocyte lineage; multiple myeloma is by far the commonest cause, accounting for three out of every five cases of paraproteinaemia (*Figure 2.1*). However, a quarter of patients have no detectable malignancy, although many have chronic disease.

Table 2.1 Monoclonal products of B lymphocyte and plasma cell tumours

Complete immunoglobulin molecules (H_2L_2)

Complete immunoglobulins (H_2L_2) and monoclonal free light chains (Bence–Jones protein)

Immunoglobulin fragments only
    Free complete light chains (Bence–Jones protein)
    Free incomplete heavy chains (heavy chain disease)
    Half-molecules (H-L)

Nonsecreting tumours

Table 2.2 Incidence of monoclonal proteins in serum

	Per cent
Blood donors (<60 years old)	0.2
Apparently healthy population	
Over 50 years old	1
Over 60 years old	2
Over 70 years old	3

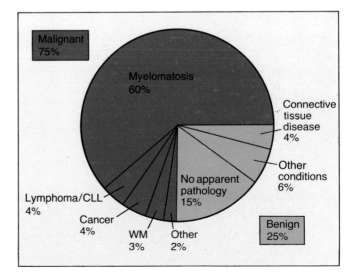

Figure 2.1 *Final diagnosis in patients with serum paraproteins of any immunoglobulin class. CLL = chronic lymphatic leukaemia; WM = Waldenström's macroglobulinaemia*

Myelomatosis

Diagnostic criteria

The Medical Research Council's criteria for the diagnosis of myelomatosis are:
(1) The demonstration of a monoclonal immunoglobulin in serum or urine.
(2) The demonstration of neoplastic monoclonal plasma cells in the bone marrow.
(3) The radiological demonstration of bone destruction.
At least two of these criteria are required to make the diagnosis.

Incidence

Myelomatosis is diagnosed with increasing frequency because of a growing awareness of its various presentations and improvements in immunochemical analysis. The incidence of the disease in Caucasians is approximately 1 per 50 000 per year but is higher in Negroes and lower in Chinese and Japanese. Myeloma is usually a disease of the elderly; the mean age at presentation is approximately 60

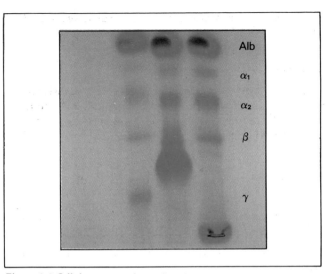

Figure 2.2 Cellulose acetate electrophoresis of sera showing the separation into albumin, α_1-. α_2-, β_1-. β_2- and γ-globulin bands. Immunoglobulins form the broad gamma band. Monoclonal proteins can be seen as discrete bands (M-bands), usually in the gamma region (IgG, IgM and IgD), although they may occur in the beta or rarely the alpha regions (IgA and free monoclonal light chains)

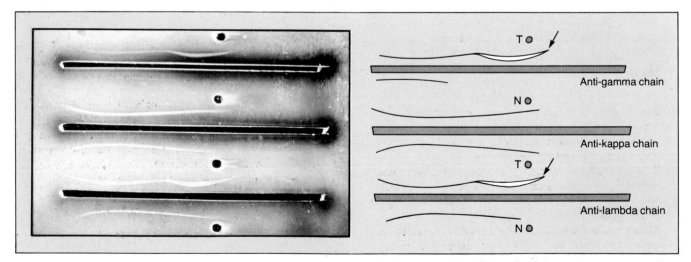

Figure 2.3 Immunoelectrophoresis in agar of test (T) and normal (N) serum. The anode is to the right. After electrophoresis, the troughs were filled with anti-gamma chain, anti-kappa light chain or anti-lambda light chain antisera. A monoclonal IgG (type lambda) is seen as a localized, thickened bowing of the relevant precipitin lines (arrowed)

years and it is uncommon below the age of 40 years. Both sexes are affected equally.

Clinical features

Presenting symptoms in patients with myelomatosis are related to either the extent of proliferation of the tumour mass or the nature or quantity of the paraprotein secreted. The appearance of a monoclonal protein may precede other manifestations by many years; thus, in about 10% of subjects, a monoclonal protein is found by chance on routine screening of serum samples or during investigation of an apparently unrelated disorder.

During the early phase, patients may be asymptomatic or complain only of nonspecific symptoms such as lethargy, malaise and weight loss. Progressive doubling of the tumour mass results in classical symptoms of established myeloma:

(1) Skeletal manifestations: tumour deposits cause bone pain, particularly in the ribs and axial skeleton. Pathological fractures are common.

(2) Hypercalcaemia: hypercalcaemia and hypercalciuria give rise to feelings of nausea, anorexia, polydipsia and polyuria.

(3) Renal impairment: renal function is usually chronically impaired in myeloma although some patients present with acute renal failure. Aetiological factors include hypercalcaemia, uric acid nephropathy, tubular precipitation of paraprotein, renal tubular acidosis, amyloidosis, pyelonephritis and drug nephrotoxicity.

(4) Bone marrow infiltration: plasma cell infiltration of the bone marrow causes anaemia and thrombocytopaenia. Suppression of normal immunoglobulin synthesis leads to recurrent pyogenic and viral infections.

(5) Vascular features: features of the hyperviscosity syndrome or cryoglobulinaemia may be clinically important in myelomatosis, although they are more usual in macroglobulinaemia.

(6) Rarer presentations: acute spinal cord compression is an uncommon presenting feature and requires emergency decompression. Amyloidosis secondary to myelomatosis can cause a carpal tunnel syndrome or peripheral neuropathy. Occasionally, patients present with skin changes such as pyoderma gangrenosum, erythema annulare, pruritus, xanthomata or yellow discoloration.

Investigations

Monoclonal immunoglobulins

Electrophoresis of serum and concentrated fresh urine will demonstrate a paraprotein in almost every case of myelomatosis (*Figure 2.2*); fewer than 1% of patients lack detectable paraprotein (that is, nonsecreting myeloma). The heavy and light chain components of the monoclonal protein can be typed by immunoelectrophoresis (*Figure 2.3*); IgG, IgA or free monoclonal light chains (Bence-Jones myeloma) account for the majority of cases (*Table 2.3*). Rarely, two distinct serum paraproteins (biclonal myeloma) can be identified in the same patient. IgM paraproteins associated with myeloma are unusual.

Table 2.3 Paraprotein type in myelomatosis

	Per cent
IgG	60
IgA	20
Light chains only	17
IgD	2
Biclonal	} 1
IgM	
IgE	(Rare)

Measurement of serum immunoglobulin concentrations is required for two reasons: first, to assess the degree of suppression of nonmyeloma immunoglobulin synthesis; and second, to measure the paraprotein level. Unfortunately, routine immunochemical methods may give misleading values, especially for IgM paraproteins. Scanning densitometric analysis of stained electrophoretic strips gives more reliable results for following the growth of the tumour.

Neoplastic plasma cells

The bone marrow shows increased numbers of abnormal plasma cells, including bi- or tri-nucleated cells with

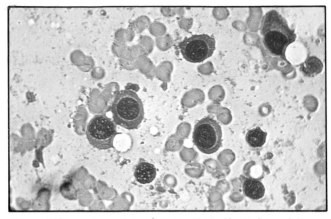

Figure 2.4 *Bone marrow from a patient with myelomatosis*

unevenly sized nuclei (*Figure 2.4*). The number of myeloma cells present is, in general, a poor guide to the progress of the disease. Although typical cases of myelomatosis show bone marrow plasmacytosis in excess of 20%, this figure can be reached in some reactive conditions and is not therefore diagnostic.

Direct immunofluorescence of bone marrow specimens using fluorescein-labelled specific antisera to heavy and light chains will confirm the monoclonal nature of the intracellular immunoglobulin and help to distinguish reactive from malignant plasmacytosis (*Figure 2.5*).

Bone destruction

Osteolytic lesions can be found in the skull in over half of all patients. The combination of osteolytic lesions and a normal serum alkaline phosphatase level is highly suggestive of myelomatosis. Generalized osteoporosis is also common but of little diagnostic value. Many patients also show compression fractures of vertebrae.

Myeloma staging by cell mass

For many tumours, careful staging of the malignancy has improved management. Durie & Salmon (1975) have shown that the myeloma cell mass at presentation correlates with survival to a clinically useful degree. They also found that certain independent factors correlated well with this calculated cell mass, which allowed them to propose a clinical staging system based on the degree of anaemia and hypercalcaemia, the extent of the osteolytic lesions and the serum concentration of the monoclonal protein (*Table 2.4*). Therapeutic response and survival are best in stage I disease (low cell mass) and worst in stage III disease (high cell mass).

Table 2.4 Myeloma staging system

	Stage I	*Stage II*	*Stage III*
Haemoglobin (g/dl)	>10.0		<8.5
Serum calcium (mmol/l)	<3.0		>3.0
(mg/dl)	<12.0		>12.0
Radiology	Normal, or one lytic lesion	Intermediate values	Lytic lesions+++
Monoclonal protein (g/l)	IgG<50 IgA<30 Urinary Bence–Jones protein <4 g/day		IgG>70 IgA>50 Urinary Bence–Jones protein >12 g/day
Myeloma cell mass ($\times 10^{12}/m^2$)	<0.6 Low cell mass	Intermediate cell mass	>1.2 High cell mass

From Durie & Salmon (1975)

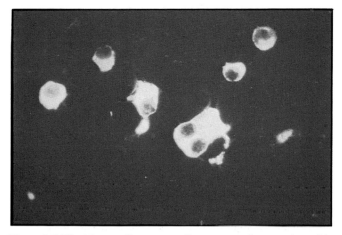

Figure 2.5 *Direct immunofluorescence of bone marrow from a patient with IgA myeloma. The marrow is incubated with a fluorescein-labelled antiserum specific for alpha chains. Dense cytoplasmic staining is seen; many of the cells also show unevenly sized nuclei or binucleated forms*

Prognostic factors

Several clinical features are of prognostic significance (*Table 2.5*). Poor renal function, defined by a raised serum creatinine level above 177 mmol/l or blood urea level above 13 mmol/l is found in approximately half of patients at presentation and is associated with a poor prognosis.

Table 2.5 Factors correlating with poor survival in myelomatosis

Raised blood urea	>13 mmol/l (>80 mg/dl)
Low serum albumin	<30 g/l
Low haemoglobin	<7.5 g/dl
Heavy Bence–Jones proteinuria	

Therapy

Induction of remission

Intermittent and continuous treatment regimes have been used; the main advantage of intermittent oral therapy is that severe marrow suppression is less common. Melpha-lan and cyclophosphamide are equally effective in inducing remission but both are toxic, particularly in the presence of renal failure. About 50–75% of patients will show a partial remission. However, most patients subsequently relapse; the median duration of remission is 9 months.

Maintenance of remission

In most patients, paraprotein levels will stop falling after 12 months, when cytotoxic treatment can be stopped to allow patients a greater feeling of wellbeing. Indeed, in one study, patients maintained beyond 12 months on various single cytotoxic drugs had no significant lengthening of survival compared with those given no maintenance therapy. Patients must, however, be closely monitored to detect relapse.

Management of relapse

When relapse occurs (*Figure 2.6*), the growth rate or doubling time of the tumour will be faster than before treatment in over 50% of cases (growth rate escape). This accelerated tumour growth is most commonly reflected in the production of Bence-Jones protein alone; occasionally there is an increased rate of synthesis of either the presenting paraprotein or another monoclonal immunoglobulin. In just under half the patients, the serum paraprotein level and by implication the myeloma cell mass grows at a rate identical to that before treatment (simple escape). Sometimes, escape from therapeutic control is due to the development of lymphoma or leukaemia.

Only 10% of relapses respond to those first-line drugs used to induce remission. The mechanism by which selective resistance to alkylating agents occurs is not known. In suitable patients, newer antitumour agents such as doxorubicin (Adriamycin) and carmustine (bischloronit-rosurea; Bicnu) may induce a further remission in about one third of cases.

Despite the use of various cytotoxic drugs, patients with multiple myeloma have a median survival period of only 2–3 years.

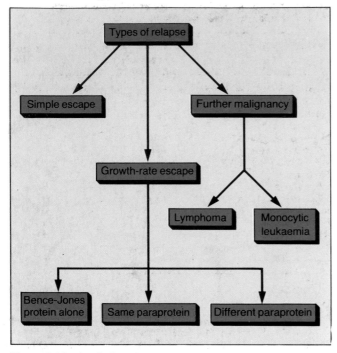

Figure 2.6 *Modes of relapse in treated cases of myelomatosis*

General care

Myeloma is a chronic disease involving many organs. While cytotoxic therapy is the definitive treatment, management of complications (*Table 2.6*) must not be overlooked. In particular, the importance of emergency treatment of hypercalcaemia and of spinal cord compression should be emphasized.

Benign monoclonal gammopathy

Benign monoclonal gammopathy can be defined as the presence of a monoclonal protein in a person showing no other manifestations of malignant disease: approximately 20–25% of all patients with paraproteins (*Figure 2.1*) have benign monoclonal gammopathy by this definition. The

Table 2.6 Management of complications of myelomatosis

Hypercalcaemia
  Rehydration
  Steroids
  Phosphate infusion
  Mithramycin

Infection
  Appropriate antibiotics
  Immunoglobulin replacement

Renal impairment
  Prevent dehydration
  Avoid fluid restriction (for example, before intravenous pyelography)
  Treat hypercalcaemia and hypercalciuria
  Standard lines of treatment

Spinal cord compression
  Laminectomy
  Localized irradiation

Hyperviscosity
  Plasmapheresis

difficulty lies in deciding whether a small amount of paraprotein in an asymptomatic subject indicates early multiple myeloma or benign monoclonal gammopathy. If no overt malignancy develops within 5 years, the paraprotein is probably benign.

Certain laboratory findings are of predictive value in distinguishing benign from malignant paraproteinaemia (*Table 2.7*). A patient with a high and increasing serum paraprotein level, suppression of normal immunoglobulin synthesis and significant Bence-Jones proteinuria is likely to develop the full clinical picture of myelomatosis within a

Table 2.7 Findings favouring malignant paraproteinaemia

1. Bence–Jones protein in serum or urine
2. Suppression of normal immunoglobulin synthesis
3. Serum paraprotein level in excess of 10 g/l
4. Rising paraprotein level with time

relatively short time. Review of all patients with paraproteinaemia at regular (3–6-monthly) intervals is therefore essential until the benign or malignant nature of the disease is established. In patients with benign monoclonal gammopathy, treatment with cytotoxic drugs is contraindicated.

IgM paraproteins

Patients with IgM serum paraproteins show a different disease distribution (*Figure 2.7*) from patients with paraproteins of any immunoglobulin class (*Figure 2.1*).

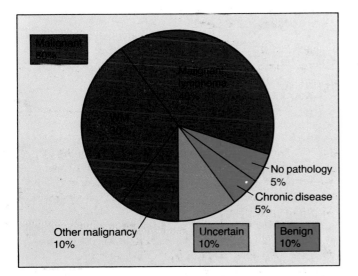

Figure 2.7 *Final diagnosis in patients with IgM class serum paraproteins. WM = Waldenström's macroglobulinaemia*

Waldenström's macroglobulinaemia

This is a slowly growing malignant tumour of lymphoid tissue in which lymphoplasmacytoid cells gradually infiltrate lymph nodes, spleen, liver and bone marrow. Unlike myeloma, symptoms of Waldenström's macroglobulinaemia (WM) (*Table 2.8*) are usually directly attributable to the effect of the monoclonal IgM on serum viscosity.

Table 2.8 Comparative clinical features of Waldenström's macroglobulinaemia and multiple myeloma

	Waldenström's macroglobulinaemia	*Multiple myeloma*
Hyperviscosity syndrome	+++	+
Changes in visual acuity	+++	+
Changes in optic fundi	+++	+
Mucosal bleeding	+++	+
Hepatosplenomegaly	+++	+
Lymphadenopathy	+++	+
Anaemia	++	+++
Neuropathy	+	+
Leucopenia		+
Thrombocytopenia		+
Renal failure		++
Hypercalcaemia		++
Recurrent infection		++
Bone pain		+++
Lytic bone lesions		+++

Clinical features

Both males and females are affected, although males predominate. The usual age at diagnosis ranges from 50 to 75 years.

There is a marked variation in the level of viscosity that produces symptoms in individual cases, but a relative serum viscosity of over 4.0 (normal 1.5 to 1.8) is usually symptomatic. Several factors contribute to the hyperviscosity syndrome (*Table 2.9*): high molecular weight paraprotein increases serum viscosity and reduces peripheral circulation; cryoglobulin precipitation causes further vascular

Table 2.9 Paraprotein characteristics contributing to the hyperviscosity syndrome

High molecular weight
High serum concentration
Confinement to the intravascular pool
Spacial configuration
Cryoglobulin formation
Adsorption to surfaces of platelets, erythrocytes and phagocytic cells

sludging, ischaemia and necrosis; and adsorption of macroglobulin to the surface of platelets, red cells and phagocytes may contribute to a bleeding tendency, anaemia and polymorph dysfunction.

On examination, the fundi show venous engorgement, haemorrhages and papilloedema. In some instances, patients present with congestive cardiac failure, hypertension, coma, cerebellar disease or epilepsy.

Investigations

Immunological findings

The characteristic abnormality is excess production of pentameric monoclonal IgM. Although free light chains may be found in urine, the concentration is usually low.

Histological findings

Bone marrow is almost invariably infiltrated by a mixture of small lymphocytes, lymphoplasmacytoid cells and plasma cells. Invasion of lymph nodes does occur but with retention of the basic node architecture. By current criteria, WM is best regarded as a low-grade lymphoplasmacytoid lymphoma.

Bone destruction

Osteolytic bone lesions and hypercalcaemia do not occur in WM.

Haematological findings

Rouleaux formation in peripheral blood smears is seen in almost all patients. Relative peripheral lymphocytosis, moderate anaemia, abnormal liver function, cold agglutinins and cryoglobulins are found in varying proportions of cases.

Treatment

Because major features of WM are due to hyperviscosity, plasmapheresis will provide rapid symptomatic relief; excess IgM is removed and the serum viscosity and plasma volume restored to normal. A plasma exchange of 2–4 litres can reduce the IgM level to 10–20% of its pretreatment level, but a more gradual effect is achieved by 1-litre exchanges daily for 5–10 days. Subsequently, maintenance plasmapheresis (1-litre exchange every 2–4 weeks) will help to keep a patient asymptomatic, provided the serum viscosity remains below 3.0.

However, plasmapheresis does nothing to retard the basic cause of the condition. Chemotherapy is therefore indicated if plasmapheresis becomes necessary more frequently than every 2–4 weeks. Chlorambucil (Leukeran) is usually given in low doses on a daily basis with frequent monitoring of blood counts.

Survival

Waldenström's macroglobulinaemia has a better prognosis than myelomatosis. Mean survival time from diagnosis is 4–5 years.

Malignant lymphoma

About 40% of IgM paraproteins are associated with lymphoma and occasionally with chronic lymphatic leukaemia. In these cases, treatment is that of the underlying condition with symptomatic relief of hyperviscosity where appropriate.

Paraproteins with antibody activity

Although the antibody specificity of most monoclonal proteins is unknown, there are many examples of paraproteins with demonstrable antibody activity.

Primary cold haemagglutinin disease

Patients with cold haemagglutinin disease (CHAD) present with a chronic haemolytic anaemia and severe Raynaud's phenomenon on exposure to cold. The associated paraprotein is nearly always IgM (type kappa); it may be a primary benign condition or arise secondary to a malignant B cell tumour (for example, lymphoma). The paraprotein reacts with components of erythrocyte membranes, usually the I antigen.

Rheumatoid factor

Paraproteins may have antibody specificity for IgG, that is, rheumatoid factor activity; they are usually IgM but monoclonal IgG and IgA rheumatoid factors can occur.

Other specificities

Rare examples of paraproteins with activity directed against factor VIII, lipoproteins or nervous tissue have been described.

Cryoglobulinaemia

Cryoglobulins are immunoglobulins which form precipitates, gels or even crystals in the cold. The clinical features are caused by simple obstruction of small blood vessels, particularly in the skin. The severity of symptoms depends on the concentration of the relevant protein and the temperature at which cryoprecipitation occurs.

Testing for cryoglobulins

Since some cryoglobulins can precipitate at temperatures above 22°C, blood should be collected in prewarmed

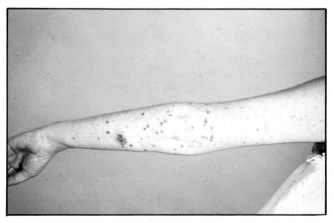

Figure 2.8 *Vasculitis with haemorrhagic blistering and ulceration in a patient with cryoglobulinaemia*

syringes and taken directly to the laboratory, where it is allowed to clot at 37°C before centrifugation. The serum is kept in a calibrated tube at 4°C for up to 72 h.

Classification

Immunoelectrophoretic analysis of cryoprecipitates allows their classification into three types:

Type I cryoglobulins (25%)

These are monoclonal proteins, usually IgM but sometimes IgG, which lack recognizable antibody specificity. They have an inherent tendency to cryoprecipitate if the protein concentration is high. In most cases, there is underlying malignant disease (usually myeloma or WM).

Symptoms result from hyperviscosity and sludging of cryoprecipitates in cutaneous vessels, producing vascular purpura (*Figure 2.8*), cutaneous ulceration and Raynaud's phenomenon.

Type II cryoglobulins (25%)

These are of mixed type, in which the monoclonal protein (usually IgM, occasionally IgG or rarely IgA) has specificity directed against the Fc portion of IgG. Cryoprecipitation occurs when complexes of IgG–anti-IgG are formed. This type is associated with lymphoma, chronic lymphatic leukaemia, macroglobulinaemia or myeloma. Patients often present with features of immune complex disease, namely diffuse vasculitis, arthritis and glomerulonephritis.

Type III cryoglobulins (50%)

These are of mixed polyclonal type in which IgM rheumatoid-like factors react with IgG. Approximately one-third of cases are idiopathic, while the remainder are associated with SLE, polyarteritis nodosa, rheumatoid arthritis and chronic infection.

Treatment

Treatment of cryoglobulinaemia is generally directed towards management of any recognized underlying disorder. Common-sense measures such as avoidance of cold environments are helpful. A combination of plasmapheresis and cytotoxic drugs can sometimes induce a remission of symptoms.

Heavy chain diseases

This rare group of diseases is characterized by the production of incomplete heavy chains without associated light chains. Three types are recognized (α-, γ- and μ-chain diseases), α-chain disease (αCD) being the most prevalent.

Alpha-chain disease

The essential abnormality is the production of incomplete α-chains by lymphoid cells infiltrating the intestinal mucosa (*Figure 2.9*). The abnormal chains can be found in serum, urine, and intestinal secretions. Most patients present with severe diarrhoea, intestinal malabsorption, weight loss, abdominal pains, and finger clubbing. The majority of cases have been described in patients from the Middle East and αCD is closely related to Mediterranean lymphoma (or immunoproliferative small intestinal disease) in its geographical, immunological and clinicopathological features. Some cases of αCD improve on antibiotic therapy alone but in others it appears to be a premalignant condition showing rapid progression to overt intestinal lymphoma. An even rarer respiratory form exists.

Gamma-chain disease

The most common presentation of gamma-chain disease resembles malignant lymphoma, with recurrent febrile episodes, painful lymphadenopathy, hepatosplenomegaly and palatal oedema. The illness is usually slowly progressive with intermittent remissions and relapses complicated by intercurrent infection.

Mu-chain disease

Small amounts of μ-chain have been described in the occasional case of otherwise typical chronic lymphatic leukaemia.

Reference

DURIE, B. G. M. and SALMON, S. E. (1975) A clinical staging system for multiple myeloma. *Cancer*, **36**, 842–854

Further reading

AMEIS, A., KO, H. S. and PRUZANSKI, W. (1976) M components – a review of 1242 cases. *Canadian Medical Association Journal*, **114**, 889–895

KHOJASTEH, A., HAGHSHENASS, M. and HAGHIGHI, P. (1983) Immunoproliferative small intestinal disease. A 'Third-World' lesion. *New England Journal of Medicine*, **308**, 1401–1405

KRAJNY, M. and PRUZANSKI, W. (1976) Waldenström's macroglobulinaemia: review of 45 cases. *Canadian Medical Association Journal*, **114**, 899–905

KYLE, R. A. (1983) Long-term survival in multiple myeloma. *New England Journal of Medicine*, **308**, 314–316

PARKER, D. and MALPAS, J. S. (1979) Multiple myeloma. *Journal of the Royal College of Physicians of London*, **13**, 146–153

WHICHER, J. T. (1983) Monoclonal proteins. In *Immunology in Medicine*, 2nd edn (E. J. Holborow and W. G. Reeves, eds). Academic Press, London

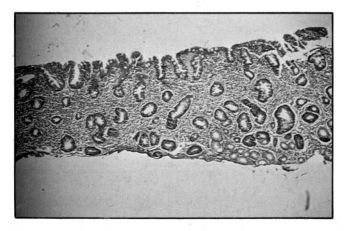

Figure 2.9 *Diffuse and extensive plasma cell infiltration of the lamina propria of the small intestine in a case of alpha-chain disease. Subtotal villous atrophy and sparsity of the crypts is apparent. Immunofluorescent studies show variable staining of the cytoplasm of these cells with anti-alpha chain antiserum but no staining with antiserum to light chains*

3   IgE and atopic disease

An important insight into the aetiology of allergic disease was the observation that allergies tend to run in families. In 1923, Coca introduced the term 'atopy', defined as a type of allergic hypersensitivity to common environmental antigens which is subject to hereditary influence. In Western countries, over 15% of the population develop some form of atopic allergic disease.

The antibody molecules initiating this response were traditionally called reagins. The major class of reaginic antibody is IgE although IgG_4 subclass antibodies possibly also make a contribution. There is now some understanding of the way in which the reaction of reaginic antibody with antigen leads to classical symptoms of acute allergic hypersensitivity. Almost everyone is endowed with the components needed to produce an allergic reaction, namely IgE (?IgG_4), mast cells, basophils, histamine and other pharmacological mediators. What is unclear is why some people never show an allergic response, why some have an

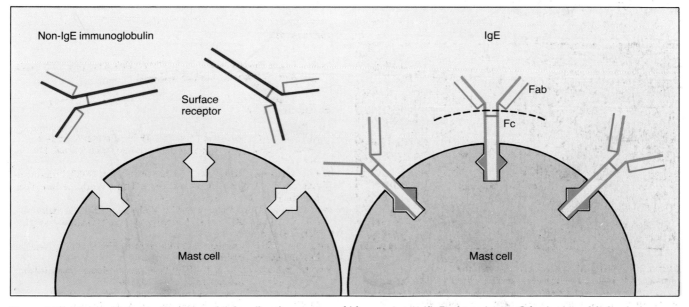

Figure 3.1 *IgE is bound to mast cells and basophils by cell surface receptors which recognize specific Fc_ϵ determinants. Other immunoglobulin classes are not bound by these receptors (with the possible exception of an IgG subclass)*

occasional mild reaction, why some suffer lifelong debilitating allergic disease, or, more rarely, why others react with severe anaphylactic shock. In view of the incomplete understanding of how an underlying atopic trait is expressed in the form of allergic symptoms, it is best to define an atopic trait as firstly, an individual tendency spontaneously to produce high levels of IgE antibodies directed against one or more common antigens and, secondly, the association of this tendency with antigen-triggered conditions in which reaginic antibody mechanisms can be identified.

Discovery of IgE

About 60 years ago, Prausnitz and Küstner demonstrated that allergic hypersensitivity could be transferred passively from one individual to another (the P-K reaction). Küstner was allergic to fish; he injected his serum intracutaneously into Prausnitz's arm and later pricked a solution of fish extract into the same area and into normal skin at a different site. A wheal and flare reaction was produced at the prepared site but not at the control site. This observation demonstrated that allergy was related to a serum factor, which was called reagin.

The isolation and description of reagin proved difficult. As each of the immunoglobulin classes was discovered, reaginic activity was mistakenly attributed to it. During the mid-1960s, Ishizaka and Ishizaka isolated a 'reagin-rich' fraction from the serum of allergic individuals, demonstrated its 'reaginic' activity, and showed that it differed immunochemically from all other known immunoglobulin classes. Because of its ability to produce erythema, they called this new immunoglobulin 'gamma E globulin'. At the same time in Sweden, Bennich and Johansson isolated a previously unknown immunoglobulin found in massive amounts in the serum of a patient with myeloma. They called this fraction immunoglobulin ND, after the patient's initials; minute amounts of IgND could block the P-K reaction, and raised levels of IgND were found in sera of patients with allergic disease. Collaborative studies soon established that IgND and gamma E globulin were the same molecule which later became recognized as the fifth class of human immunoglobulin and officially designated immunoglobulin E (IgE).

IgE molecule

Structure

IgE has the Y-shaped structure common to all classes of immunoglobulin (see Chapter 1). The Fab fragments enclose the antigen-binding sites and the Fc portion contains the determinants that make IgE a unique class.

Biological properties

The serum concentration of IgE is minute, generally in the nanogram range. However, the bulk of IgE in any individual is bound to the surface membranes of circulating basophils and tissue mast cells, as a result of surface receptors recognizing determinants in the Fc portion of the ϵ-chain of IgE. The IgE bound to the target-cell surface is presumed to present its antigen-binding sites (Fab regions) to the microenvironment of the cell (*Figure 3.1*) and is thus still able to react with specific antigen. The number of Fc_ϵ receptors on human basophils is approximately 40 000 to 100 000 per cell, although not all receptor sites are necessarily occupied by IgE molecules. The binding of IgE molecules by basophils and mast cells is very strong; this high affinity compensates for the low serum levels of IgE and its rapid catabolism (half-life: 2 days), allowing the biological activity of cell-bound IgE to persist much longer than in the free state. Paradoxically, this persistence may be deleterious to an atopic person.

There is no evidence that, in the atopic individual, IgE is bound more avidly to target-cell receptor sites than in the nonatopic person. The elevated level of serum IgE in the atopic population is related to increased synthesis and means that target-cell receptor sites of atopic individuals are likely to be more highly saturated than those of normal people.

Additional information on the biological properties of IgE is shown in Chapter 1 (*Tables 1.1 and 1.2*).

Triggering of mediator release

It is generally accepted that the release of biologically active mediators is triggered when an antigen molecule interacts with two adjacent cell-bound IgE antibody molecules, so forming a bridge composed of IgE–antigen–IgE (*Figure 3.2*). This implies that the antigen must possess repeating antigenic sites per molecule, with a minimum of two sites. This interaction induces conformational changes in the target-cell surface membrane, activating intracellular enzyme systems and culminating in the release of the mediators of acute hypersensitivity. However, mediator release can also be induced by preformed IgE–antigen complexes, polymerized IgE without antigen, Fc fragments of IgE and by anti-IgE antibodies, suggesting that antigen is not always required for mediator release. More recently, it has been shown that the Fc_ϵ receptors on the cell surface and their bound IgE molecules migrate as a complex on the cell membrane. Bridging of cell-bound IgE molecules will also bring these receptor sites into close proximity. Mediator release from mast cells can be triggered by antisera raised against the exposed regions of the IgE receptor sites (*Figure 3.2*) and by the $F(ab')_2$ fragments of these antisera, but not by the Fab fragments, implying that bridging of a pair of receptor molecules is primarily responsible for the activation of membrane-associated enzymes.

Non-IgE triggered release of mediators can cause clinically relevant disease: some known nonimmune factors include naturally occurring endogenous substances (such as acetylcholine, α-adrenergic substances, prostaglandins and complement components) and exogenous chemicals and drugs which act by poorly understood mechanisms. For example, in recent years, immediate anaphylactic-like reactions have been reported following the administration of several intravenous anaesthetic agents, radiocontrast media and plasma volume expanders. In most instances, prior exposure to the drug is not required and IgE antibodies are not involved. The most likely explanation is that such agents either directly activate the complement system with release of the complement-derived anaphylatoxic fragments C3a and C5a (see Chapter 4) or directly trigger basophils and/or mast cells.

In most if not all allergic individuals, there is some degree of nonimmune triggering in addition to the classical IgE-mediated release of chemical mediators.

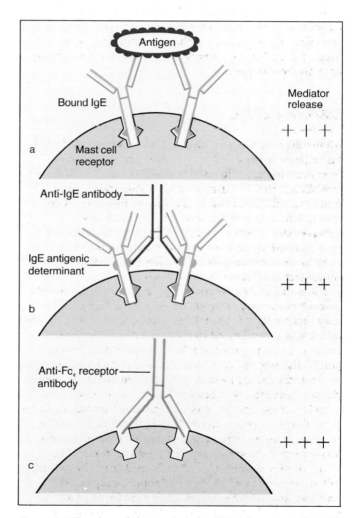

Figure 3.2 *The release of pharmacological mediators from mast cells and basophils can be triggered not only by specific antigen* (a) *but also by antisera to cell-bound IgE* (b) *or the surface receptors* (c)

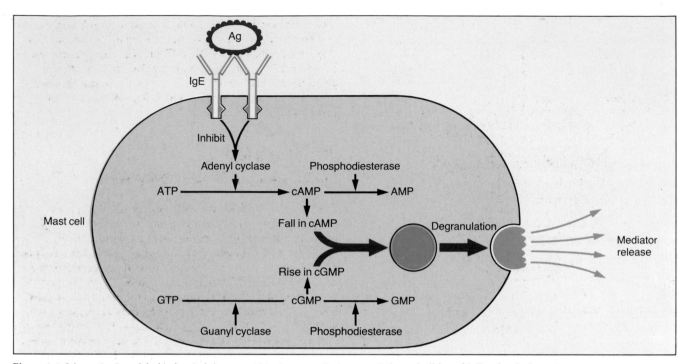

Figure 3.3 *Schematic view of the biochemical changes within the mast cell after cross-linkage of cell-bound IgE molecules by antigen*

Effects of mediators

Mast cells and basophils respond to an extracellular or cell-membrane-bound first messenger which operates through an intracellular second messenger. The first message comes from the cross-linking, by antigen, of IgE-receptor complexes on the cell surface and the second comes from adenyl cyclase, an enzyme that generates cyclic AMP (cyclic 3′, 5′-adenosine monophosphate) from adenosine triphosphate (ATP) (*Figure 3.3*). Combination of antigen with IgE inhibits adenyl cyclase, producing a fall in cyclic AMP to a critical level; the granules are transported to the cell membrane and discharged. Mediators liberated from mast cells and basophils may be *preformed* (that is, present in cytoplasmic granules ready for release) or *newly generated* (that is, synthesized following the triggering stimulus and after the release of preformed mediators).

Preformed mediators are histamine, lysosomal enzymes, neutrophil chemotactic factor (NCF), eosinophil chemotactic factor of anaphylaxis (ECF-A) and heparin. Other mediators are newly generated from arachidonic acid via the cyclo-oxygenase and lipoxygenase pathways: these include prostaglandins (especially PGD_2), thromboxanes, leukotrienes (LT) and platelet activating factor (PAF). It has been shown recently that slow-reacting substance of anaphylaxis (SRS-A) is composed of a mixture of LT C4, LT D4 and LT E4. These mediators all contribute to the variable clinical features of acute hypersensitivity (*Figure 3.4*). Furthermore, indirect activation of the complement pathway and the coagulation and fibrinolytic systems can further generate additional components with similar biological effects. There are considerable species differences in the relative importance of these different mediators and their target organ susceptibilities. In humans, the respira-

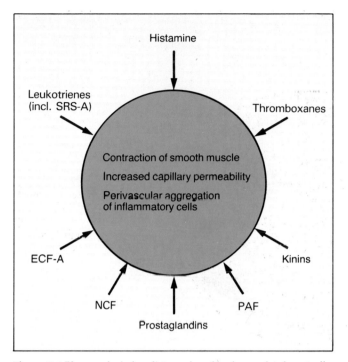

Histamine

Leukotrienes (incl. SRS-A)

Thromboxanes

Contraction of smooth muscle

Increased capillary permeability

Perivascular aggregation of inflammatory cells

ECF-A

Kinins

NCF

PAF

Prostaglandins

Figure 3.4 *Pharmacological mediators released by degranulated mast cells and basophils*

tory and vascular systems are most affected by acute IgE-mediated reactions.

It has long been known that a 'delayed' reaction can occur following mast cell degranulation. This late phase response begins 4–6 h after the initial reaction, peaks around 12 h and last 24–36 h. Such late responses are incompletely understood, but are IgE-dependent and most frequently affect the lung and skin.

Other mast cell sensitizing antibodies

Although IgE is the main and best known mast cell sensitizing antibody there is evidence that a subclass of IgG, probably IgG_4, is also capable of passively sensitizing mast cells in man. In contrast to IgE, which is heat-labile and able to sensitize mediator cells for up to several weeks,

IgG_4 is heat-stable and capable of sensitization for only a few hours. There is limited but growing evidence that this short-term sensitizing (STS) IgG antibody is implicated in several clinical situations, for example, extrinsic allergic alveolitis in bird fanciers, and asthma due to the house dust mite. Of course, both IgE and STS–IgG antibodies may occur in the same individual.

Biological role of IgE

Unusual features of the IgE antibody system

Certain aspects of IgE antibody synthesis are unusual compared with other immunoglobulin classes. First, IgE antibodies are present only in minute amounts in the serum; this is true even in atopic individuals, although their circulating levels may be many thousand times higher than normal. Second, IgE is synthesized locally in the respiratory and gastrointestinal mucosa, suggesting an important role for such antibodies in protecting the host against agents likely to invade at these sites. Third, the antigens which readily stimulate IgE production differ in some ways from antigens stimulating responses of other immunoglobulin classes: for example, parasitic nematodes usually induce high titres of IgE antibodies whereas bacteria and viruses usually stimulate high titres of IgM and IgG antibodies but not IgE.

Role of IgE in parasite expulsion

It has been known for many years that parasite infestation results in production of very high levels of IgE. Several lines of evidence suggest that parasite-specific IgE antibodies play a significant part in the protection of the infected host. First, a positive correlation exists between the ability to produce IgE antibodies and the degree of effective immunity against *Schistosoma mansoni*. Second, macrophages possess receptors for IgE molecules; cross-linkage of IgE molecules by parasite antigens activates macrophages and induces the release of lysosomal enzymes. Third, IgE antibodies foster immune adherence of normal macrophages (from experimental animals) to *S. mansoni* schistosomules, the adhered macrophages readily killing attached organisms.

It is also possible that IgE-mediated release of inflammatory mediators from intestinal mast cells participates directly in the expulsion of parasites from the gut, so reducing the parasitic load. Interestingly, the high level of IgE in patients with helminthic infestation is not associated with an increased frequency of allergic disease; common atopic conditions such as asthma are less common in tropical populations endemically infected with parasites. It has been suggested that the emergence of clinical forms of atopic disease in more highly developed countries is the price we pay for a reduction in our parasitic load.

Regulation of IgE antibody synthesis

IgE levels and age

IgE is rarely detectable in the cord blood of human neonates because IgE synthesis is not 'switched on' in utero under normal circumstances. Following birth, however, serum IgE levels show some unusual characteristics. Mean serum IgE rises steadily throughout childhood, reaching a peak in early adolescence which is higher than mean adult levels: between 12 and 20 years of age, levels fall to the adult mean, followed by a further slow fall after the age of 60 years. IgE also has a much wider normal range than is found for other immunoglobulin classes.

Hereditary aspects of allergic disease

Although allergies tend to 'run in families', many studies of the inheritance of allergic disease have shown that it is not controlled by a single gene behaving in a strict mendelian dominant or recessive pattern. Nevertheless, the family history can often be used to assess the risk of developing allergic disease (*Figure 3.5*). Even a child whose parents have no history of allergic symptoms still has approximately a one in eight chance of developing allergic disease sometime during his or her lifetime.

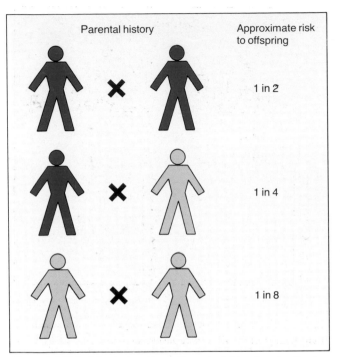

Figure 3.5 *Risk of developing allergic disease in children born to allergic or nonallergic parents (allergic parents are shown in red)*

Genetic control

Different strains of laboratory animals vary greatly in their capacity to produce IgE antibody after specific immunization (*Figure 3.6*). Most strains require a large dose of antigen to produce an IgE response which, when it occurs, is transient and usually cannot be boosted by further antigenic exposure – a situation rather analogous to nonatopic humans. In contrast, certain strains develop unusually high levels of IgE antibody following immunization with small doses of antigen and are capable of producing secondary responses as well, a situation similar to the atopic state in man.

In the mouse, the capacity to develop high titres of persistent IgE antibody to an antigen is genetically controlled and linked to the MHC situated on chromosome 17. Genes specifically controlling immune responses to

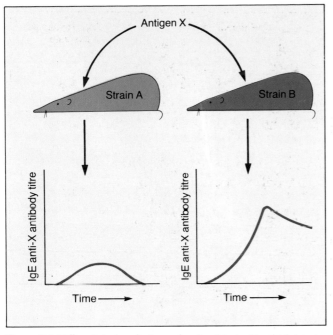

Figure 3.6 *Different strains of mice produce low (strain A) or high (strain B) titres of specific IgE antibodies after immunization with antigen X*

individual antigens are termed Ir genes and genes determining high responsiveness are dominant over those coding for low responsiveness to the same antigen. A strain which is a high responder to one antigen, however, may be a low responder to a different, unrelated antigen. In humans, it has been postulated that analogous Ir genes also exist, linked to the major histocompatibility (HLA) complex on chromosome 6. Evidence suggests that one such Ir gene controls the immune response to ragweed antigen E: thus, segregation analysis of two large families with atopic disease indicated autosomal dominant inheritance of seasonal ragweed allergy, the locus for this trait being HLA-linked.

Regulation of IgE antibody synthesis by T lymphocytes

Rats which normally produce high-titre IgE antibodies following immunization with an appropriate antigen

(*Figure 3.7*) cannot do so if they are subjected to neonatal thymectomy before immunization. This defect can be overcome by supplementation of thymectomized animals with normal thymocytes (*Figure 3.7*), showing that thymus-derived lymphocytes are needed for the development of an IgE antibody response. Furthermore, cooperation between both T and B lymphocytes is essential for the synthesis of specific IgE antibodies. This can be demonstrated in an adoptive cell transfer system (*Figure 3.8*): heavy irradiation of mice eliminates most of the lymphoid cells and prevents the mice from making a natural immune response. If the

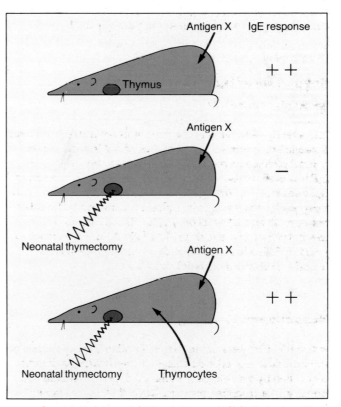

Figure 3.7 *The effect of neonatal thymectomy on the synthesis of specific IgE antibody to antigen X. Failure to produce IgE after thymectomy can be overcome by supplementing thymectomized animals with normal thymocytes. This demonstrates the need for thymus-derived lymphocytes in the IgE antibody response*

mice are inoculated with normal lymphocyte subpopulations together with an appropriate antigen, it is apparent that cooperation between T and B lymphocytes is necessary for IgE antibody production (*Figure 3.8*). By using cells with an identifiable chromosome marker, plasma cells can be shown exclusively to secrete the IgE antibodies, yet the presence of T cells is essential to allow B cells to develop into IgE plasma cells.

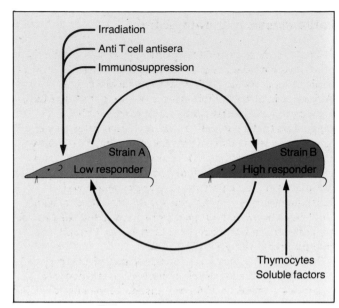

Figure 3.9 *Experimental procedures capable of converting mice from low IgE-responder strains into high-responder animals: evidence that the regulation of IgE synthesis is normally limited by a suppressor mechanism*

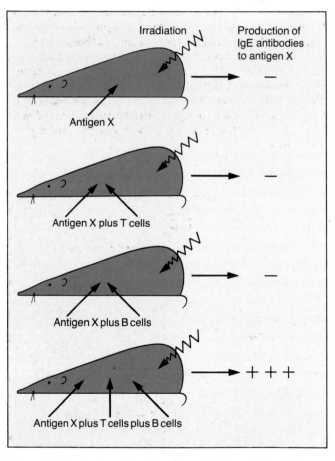

Figure 3.8 *The adoptive cell transfer system: the demonstration that cooperation between T and B lymphocytes is needed for the production of specific IgE antibodies*

While these studies illustrate the need for T lymphocyte participation in IgE antibody responses, the more intriguing question is what mechanisms normally prevent or minimize the development of excessive IgE antibody synthesis in strains of animals belonging to the low IgE responder phenotype. These strains do not have an innate incapacity to respond since experimental manipulations, such as appropriate doses of whole body irradiation, administration of some anti-T-cell antisera or certain immunosuppressive drugs can convert these animals from low to high IgE production (*Figure 3.9*). The enhanced IgE responder animals can be converted back to poor responders by the passive transfer of T cells from normal littermates or by soluble factors derived from these cells. The implication is that regulation of IgE antibody synthesis is dominated by a suppressor T cell regulatory or 'damping' mechanism which limits the extent of IgE antibody production following antigen sensitization.

Pathogenesis of the atopic trait

Several theories attempt to explain why some individuals produce IgE antibodies to common environmental antigens while others do not. The increased incidence of IgA deficiency in atopic individuals and an increased incidence of atopy in IgA-deficient subjects have lead to the suggestion that a qualitative or quantitative deficiency of IgA at mucosal surfaces allows the absorption of excessive amounts of antigens capable of stimulating IgE synthesis. The observation of a transient period of IgA deficiency in the infants of atopic parents and its association with subsequent onset of symptoms would support this theory. However, the experimental work in animals outlined above suggests a different concept which has been termed 'allergic breakthrough' by Katz (1980).

This concept (*Figure 3.10*) considers that IgE production is normally kept at a low level following sensitization by a damping mechanism which reflects the net balance of the suppressive versus enhancing regulatory factors involved. If, when some disturbance depresses the damping capacity beyond a critical level, the individual is simultaneously exposed to one or more appropriate antigens, the allergic breakthrough could result in excessive IgE antibody production to the relevant antigens and the subsequent development of symptoms. In addition, one must also consider the genetic predisposition of any individual to be capable of responding to the antigens concerned.

In children, onset or exacerbation of allergic disease often follows a viral respiratory infection. It is possible that upper respiratory tract infections are a common although transient cause of perturbation of the damping mechanism by selectively affecting T suppressor cells. In one prospective study, the onset of clinical and immunological evidence of allergy in children of allergic parents usually coincided with, or closely followed upper respiratory tract infection, most commonly with parainfluenza virus or respiratory syncytial virus.

27

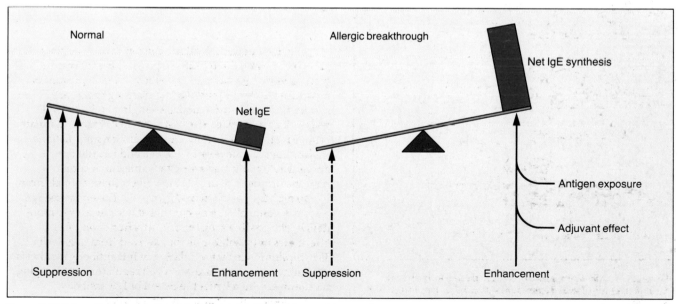

Figure 3.10 *Schematic representation of the 'allergic breakthrough' concept (see text for explanation)*

Diagnostic tools in the investigation of allergic disease

Clues from the history and examination

A detailed history should suggest a provisional diagnosis and indicate the most suitable procedures needed to confirm this diagnosis. Two important questions are whether allergic symptoms are seasonal or perennial and whether they are worse indoors or outdoors.

Seasonal allergies in the UK are usually caused by pollens and, in general, trees pollinate first, followed by grasses and then weeds. Moulds sporulate during the grass and weed pollen season; this may cause diagnostic difficulty since moulds occur on both indoor and outdoor plants. Perennial allergies are most likely to be caused by house-dust mite, foods, animals and yeasts.

Although a family history of atopic disease will reinforce other evidence of an atopic trait it will not provide any clue as to the specific sensitivities of the patient under investigation.

Total IgE levels

A raised serum IgE level provides an objective measure of an atopic state but gives no pointer as to the cause of the symptoms. IgE levels will, however, help to identify the patient at risk, whether or not he or she is symptomatic. While many variables other than IgE contribute to the clinical features of allergy in adults or older children, the serum IgE level alone may be a helpful diagnostic and prognostic tool during the first two years of life: at this early age, the distinction between atopic and nonatopic individuals is much clearer. In the atopic child the serum IgE level rises earlier and climbs higher than in normal children. Total serum IgE levels can therefore be of value in infants with a positive family history of atopic disease and in infants with troublesome symptoms of suspected allergic origin.

The diagnostic value of serum IgE determinations in adults and older children is less clear-cut. High serum IgE levels often accompany atopic disease, particularly asthma, seasonal allergic rhinitis and atopic eczema. The levels seem, in general, to be related to antigen exposure; the

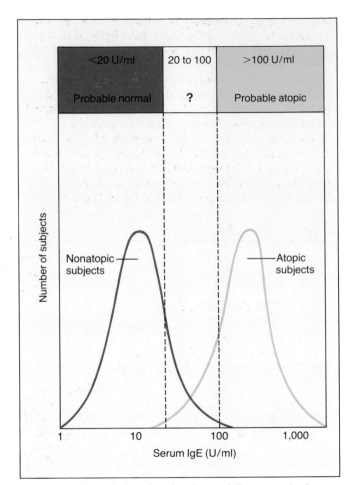

Figure 3.11 *The predictive value of total serum IgE concentration in distinguishing atopic from nonatopic adults*

longer the period of exposure and the more antigens the patient is sensitive to, then the higher the IgE level.

Serum IgE levels show a wide variation (*Figure 3.11*). Some 'normal' individuals may have raised IgE levels while, conversely, a low serum IgE does not preclude an allergic aetiology. Occasional patients are sensitive to one antigen: as a result, total IgE may be normal while skin tests or radio allergosorbent tests (see below) are positive.

Nevertheless, approximately two-thirds of nonatopic subjects and only 2% of atopic patients have IgE levels below 20 U/ml. In contrast, almost two-thirds of the atopic patients have levels in excess of 100 U/ml (*Figure 3.11*).

Serum IgE concentrations are also raised in nonatopic conditions (*Figure 3.12*), particularly parasitic infestation and quoted 'normal' ranges for Europeans may not apply to residents from zones where parasites are endemic.

Measurement of the total IgE level is not essential in any clinical condition; instead it should be considered a rough diagnostic tool, most useful when the clinical picture is ambiguous or other test results are difficult to evaluate. In clinically convincing cases of allergy, the test adds nothing.

Radio allergosorbent tests

The most widely used technique for detecting and measuring antigen-specific IgE antibodies is the radio allergosorbent test (RAST: Pharmacia Diagnostics). The RAST procedure is simple (*Figure 3.13*). A paper disc labelled with antigen is incubated with a small amount of test serum. After washing the disc to remove free unbound IgE, radiolabelled anti-human IgE is added. After further washing to remove free, unbound, radioactive label, the level of radioactivity attached to the disc is measured, the amount of antigen-specific IgE being directly related to the counts obtained. The use of a specific antiserum to human

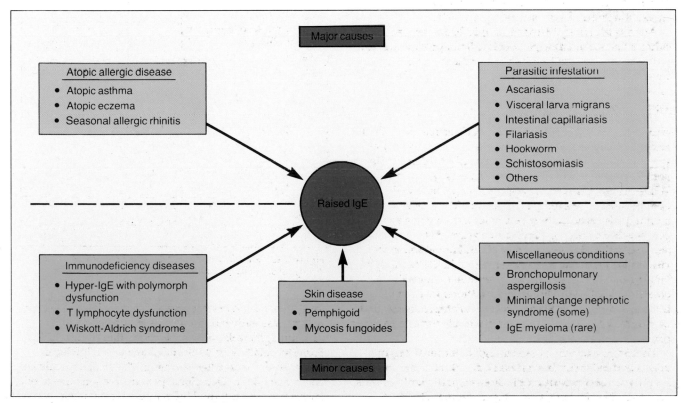

Figure 3.12 *Principal causes of elevated serum IgE*

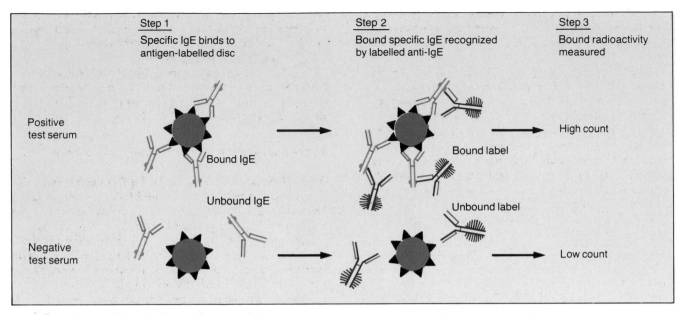

Figure 3.13 *Principle of the radio allergosorbent test*

IgE means that antibodies of other immunoglobulin classes are not recognized in this assay.

RAST results are interpreted by comparison with a reference sample run in parallel and classified as negative (class 0), borderline (1), positive (2), strongly positive (3) or very strongly positive (4).

The diagnostic value of RAST is often assessed by comparison with skin testing and nasal or bronchial provocation tests. While the overall agreement between RAST and such tests is about 75–85%, agreement is higher in patients with moderate to severe hypersensitivity but considerably lower for milder hypersensitivity. The usual type of discordance between tests *in vitro* and *in vivo* is a positive RAST with a negative skin or provocation test. In most cases, the mild degree of hypersensitivity detected by RAST is of doubtful clinical importance. In some cases, however, a negative RAST is found in a patient with positive skin or provocation tests, highlighting the danger in assuming that serum IgE specificities necessarily reflect those of tissue-fixed IgE.

RAST assays are expensive and time-consuming: most laboratories are rightly unwilling to screen sera against a large panel of antigens indiscriminately. Skin testing is a cheaper and quicker way of identifying those antigens to which the patient can mount an IgE-mediated reaction. RAST testing need only be performed when skin testing is unreliable or contraindicated: for example, in very young children; in patients with severe and extensive eczema or dermographism; in those in whom symptomatic treatment may influence skin reactions; in patients with exceptionally high levels of sensitization in whom even skin testing is potentially hazardous; and in some patients with 'food allergy' where skin testing may be unreliable. Properly used, RAST testing can reduce the frequency of provocation tests.

Skin tests

Prick testing is a traditional and sensitive diagnostic tool in allergic disease. The assumption is made that skin responsiveness reflects and correlates with the reactivity of the mucous membranes of the bronchi, nose and other target organs. However, there is no clear evidence that this is so.

Many factors can affect prick test reactivity (*Figure 3.14*). Variability in the potency of antigen extracts may be considerable among batches from different suppliers or even in lots from the same source. Differences in the stability and purity of extracts also affect biological potency, and the preservatives used to improve stability and prevent contamination, for example phenol, can have nonspecific irritant effects. The magnitude and reproducibility of the response is often influenced by the biological variability of the skin. In healthy individuals, skin reactivity is greatest at about the third decade and declines from the fifth decade onwards; skin reactivity may vary with circadian rhythms and menstrual cycles and, in the presence of dermographism there will be positive skin tests to all antigens, including negative saline controls.

Despite these hazards, clinical studies have shown that prick tests provide good specificity (few false positives) and good sensitivity (few false negatives) in patients with moderate or high degrees of sensitization.

Basophil degranulation and histamine release tests

Human basophils which have fixed IgE antibodies will degranulate on the addition of specific antigen: degranulation can be scored morphologically or by measuring histamine release. In practice, basophils from a normal (nonallergic) individual or animal cell preparations (rat mast cells, chopped monkey lung) are passively sensitized with serum from an allergic patient. Although the method is reliable when performed with appropriate controls by experienced investigators, present application of the method is limited by the need for large volumes of fresh blood (or animal tissue) to provide sufficient numbers of functioning basophils.

Provocation tests *in vivo*

Target organ challenge with a suspected antigen is, in theory, the best test of allergy because it most closely simulates the physiological effect of natural exposure. As routine clinical procedures, however, provocation tests are of limited value because they are time-consuming, affected by the medication being taken by the patient, and cannot be used in a symptomatic patient.

In the case of bronchial provocation tests, a major source of misleading results is the tendency of some patients with hyper-reactive airways to respond to numerous nonimmunological stimuli such as impurities or preservatives in the antigen extracts.

Nasal challenge is useful in patients with a history suggestive of allergic rhinitis. Some patients have negative RAST or skin tests yet show positive reactions to nasal challenge, reflecting the ill-defined nature of these antigens

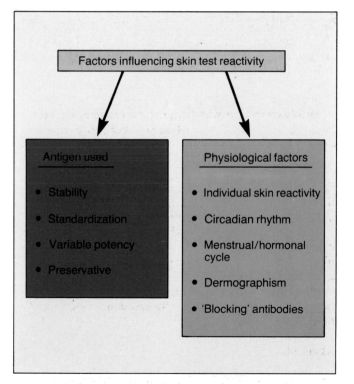

Figure 3.14 *Factors influencing skin test reactivity*

and the varying potencies of available extracts. Specific IgE antibodies can be demonstrated sometimes in the nasal secretions. Major problems with nasal provocation tests include their lack of value if the nasal mucosa is already congested, or if the patient is taking medication, the subjective nature of the criteria required for a positive result and the need to limit testing to one antigen at a time.

Food allergy often presents a difficult diagnostic problem. A high index of clinical suspicion is required since skin tests with dietary antigens, total IgE levels and RAST often fail to correlate with the clinical picture. A diagnosis of food allergy can be confirmed only by observation of symptomatic relief on dietary withdrawal of the offending food and the return of symptoms following food challenge.

Therapeutic approaches in the management of allergic disease

Several therapeutic manoeuvres are possible in the management of allergic disease (*Figure 3.15*).

Antigen avoidance

Where possible, elimination of the offending antigen, for example animal dander, constitutes the simplest and most effective form of treatment. Unfortunately for most sufferers, environmental antigens are difficult to avoid.

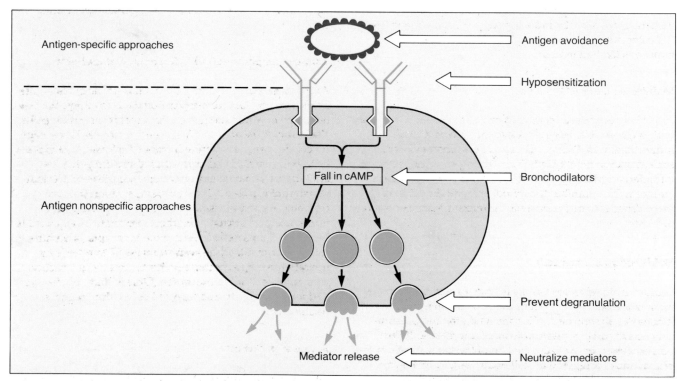

Figure 3.15 *Therapeutic manoeuvres in the management of allergic disease and their possible sites of action*

Neutralization of binding of antigen to cell-bound IgE

'Hyposensitization' procedures are based on repeated injections of increasing amounts of specific antigen spaced over a period of weeks. Initial doses of antigen extracts must be insufficient to trigger an immediate hypersensitivity reaction. Success in hyposensitization is usually attributed to the stimulation of IgG antibodies which combine with circulating antigen and 'block' the reaction of antigen with IgE-coated mast cells. Although treated patients often show a rise in IgG and a fall in IgE levels during hyposensitization procedures, there is little correlation between the titre of 'blocking' antibody and the degree of clinical improvement. In experimental animals, it is a critical requirement for good IgE responses that the immunizing dose of antigen is very small. Persistent immunization, or high doses of antigen, can abrogate this response, probably by inducing suppressor T cell activity. A similar mechanism may explain the response to hyposensitization in man.

Maintenance of cAMP levels

As already discussed, combination of antigen with cell-bound IgE inhibits adenyl cyclase, producing a fall in intracellular cAMP levels. Beta$_2$-adrenergic stimulators such as salbutamol, terbutaline and orciprenaline, stimulate adenyl cyclase activity. Xanthine derivatives, such as aminophylline, inhibit phosphodiesterase: the effect of these drugs is to maintain a high intracellular concentration of cAMP.

Stabilization of mast cells

Sodium cromoglycate (Intal) has transformed the management of allergic disease yet its mode of action is not known. It does not directly neutralize any mediator and presumably acts at some point prior to mediator release. It does not, however, prevent the fixation of IgE to mast cells or the interaction of antigen with cell-bound antibody. It is not steroid-like and acts independently of adrenergic or cholinergic pathways. The predominant mode of action is thought to be the stabilization of mast cell membranes although an inhibitory effect on phosphodiesterase has been postulated also.

Although the administration of systemic corticosteroids often produces dramatic relief of symptoms in severe asthma and the introduction of potent steroid aerosols (for example, beclomethasone, Becotide) has reduced the problem of adrenal suppression, their mode of action in reversing airways obstruction is still poorly understood. One of the major pharmacological functions of corticosteroids is to stabilize biomembranes against rupture by a variety of agents. However, they are probably not effective in blocking the IgE-mediated release of histamine from mast cells. It seems more likely therefore that corticosteroids act either by diminishing the clinical effects of released mediators, or by inhibiting the release of arachidonic acid from cell membranes and hence the generation of some mediators.

Pharmacological neutralization of mediator effects

Antihistames competitively inhibit the effects of histamine by blocking histamine receptors on nerve endings, but have no effect on histamine release from mast cells or basophils. The competitive action of histamine analogues is best seen when they are given before histamine release. As this must be the case rarely in allergic states, these drugs have a limited role in the management of atopic disease. Certain nonsteroidal anti-inflammatory drugs inhibit the cyclo-oxygenase enzyme responsible for prostaglandin and thromboxane formation and therefore might be expected to inhibit reactions in which these mediators play a dominant role. Experimental drugs can suppress LT synthesis by inhibiting the lipoxygenase pathway: this mode of action was proposed for benoxaprofen (Opren), but no selective anti-allergic activity was reported before the drug was withdrawn.

Future approaches

The most logical approach to the therapy of allergic disease is to prevent or suppress the production of IgE antibodies following stimulation by common environmental antigens. From basic research into the regulation of the immune system in general, and the control of IgE synthesis in particular, have come new insights with implications for the future treatment of IgE-mediated disorders. One advance has been the recognition that Ir genes, linked to the MHC, may control the specific responses to some antigens. Identification of such genes and their products in humans may allow prediction of individuals at risk – that is, those who are genetically high IgE responders to any given antigen. The recognition that IgE antibody production is normally damped by suppressor T cell mechanisms suggests that selective suppressor factors derived from these cells could in future be used to inhibit IgE antibody synthesis.

Reference

KATZ, D. H. (1980) Recent studies on the regulation of IgE antibody synthesis in experimental animals and man. *Immunology*, **41**, 1–24

Further reading

EDITORIAL (1983) Inflammatory mediators of asthma. *Lancet*, **2**, 829–831

FLETCHER, M. and GERSHWIN, E. (1983) Insights into mast-cell biology and IgE production. *Immunology Today*, **4**, 305–306

HOLGATE, S. T. and KAY, A. B. (1984) Mast cells and the lung. *Hospital Update*, **10**, 151–162

ISHIZAKA, T. and ISHIZAKA, K. (1975) Biology of immunoglobulin E. Molecular basis of reaginic hypersensitivity. *Progress in Allergy*, **19**, 60–121

LEWIS, R. A. and AUSTEN, K. F. (1981) Mediation of local homeostasis and inflammation by leukotrienes and other mast-cell-dependent compounds. *Nature (London)*, **293**, 103–106

REEVES, W. G. (1983) Atopic disorders. In *Immunology in Medicine*, 2nd edn (E. J. Holborow and W. G. Reeves, eds). Academic Press, London

ROYAL COLLEGE OF PHYSICIANS AND THE BRITISH NUTRITION FOUNDATION (1984) Food intolerance and food aversion. *Journal of the Royal College of Physicians of London*, **18**, 83–123

WORLD HEALTH ORGANIZATION (1981) Use and abuse of laboratory tests in clinical immunology: critical considerations of eight widely used diagnostic procedures. *Clinical and Experimental Immunology*, **46**, 662–674

4 Complement and disease

Definition of complement

Complement is a complex series of interacting plasma proteins which form a major effector system for antibody-mediated immune reactions. The results of complement activation include increased vascular permeability, attraction of leucocytes, enhanced phagocytosis and cell lysis. Lysis occurs only when all components react: however, other vital biological properties are attributable to some of the intermediate complexes.

Terminology

Complement components are numbered in order of activation. The exception is C4, which was the fourth component described but is now known to act second in the sequence. Activated components are shown with a bar over the number – for example C1 is activated to $\overline{C1}$ – and fragments by letters after the number – for example C3 is split into two fragments C3a and C3b. In addition, specific inhibitors of certain components are designated according to their site of action, for example C1 inhibitor or C3b inactivator (also called factor I).

Principles of complement activation

Complement components normally exist as inactive precursors: activation often involves limited proteolytic cleavage of the component into two or more fragments (*Figure 4.1*). One fragment possesses both a *binding* site for attachment

to cell membranes or to the initiating immune complex and an *enzymatic* site for cleavage of the next component in the sequence. However, only a proportion of any activated molecules become cell-bound, the remainder being re-

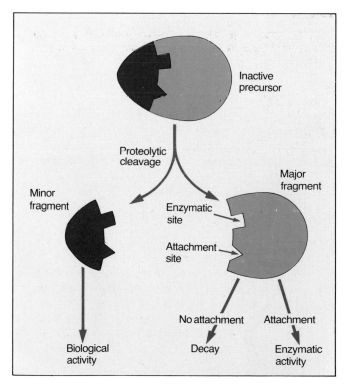

Figure 4.1 *Basic principles underlying the cleavage of complement components*

35

leased into the surrounding fluid where they decay naturally or are specifically inactivated. Since their functional properties cannot be regenerated, inactivated fragments do not participate further in the complement sequence. This rapid decay and inhibition of active sites ensures that potentially harmful effects are confined to the initiating antigen without involving bystander host cells.

The second or subsequent fragments generated by the cleavage of a component may have important biological properties in the fluid phase, such as chemotactic activity.

Complement activation pathways

Complement activation occurs in two distinct but overlapping phases (*Figure 4.2*); activation of the C3 component followed by activation of the 'attack' sequence. The critical step is the cleavage of C3 by complement-derived enzymes termed 'C3 convertases'. This generates a major fragment C3b which fixes to the initiating immune complexes and promotes their adherence to receptors on phagocytic and other cells, so amplifying the biological effects of complement activation.

The cleavage of C3 is achieved via two routes, the 'classical' and 'alternative' pathways, both of which generate C3 convertases but in response to different stimuli.

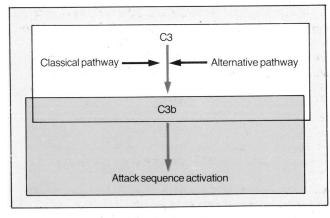

Figure 4.2 *Simplified view of complement activation. The boxes represent the two distinct but overlapping phases*

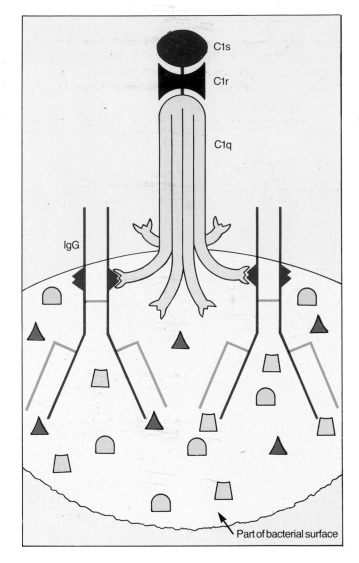

Figure 4.3 *Classical pathway activation: C1q reacts with exposed binding sites (shown in red) in the Fc region of IgG or IgM antibodies which have reacted with the specific antigenic determinants (shown in brown, green and violet) characterizing the surface of a microorganism*

Classical pathway activation

C1, the first protein in the sequence, is itself a complex of three subcomponents, C1q, C1r and C1s, held together by calcium ions. C1q is a remarkable, collagen-like protein composed of six subunits (*Figure 4.3*), resembling a 'bunch

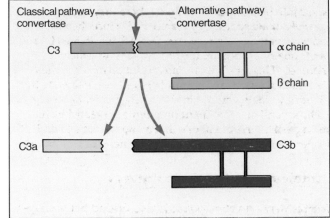

Figure 4.5 *C3 component: classical and alternative pathway C3 convertases split C3 at the same site on the α chain, generating C3a and C3b fragments*

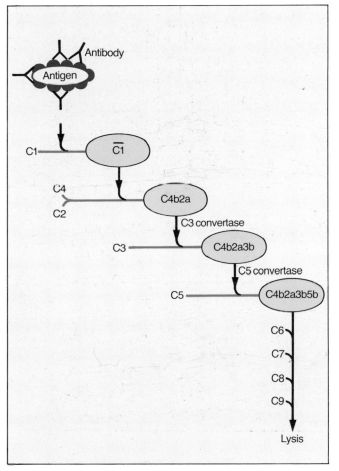

Figure 4.4 *Classical pathway activation: the complement cascade resulting from C1 binding by the appropriate antigen–antibody reaction and culminating in lytic activity. Intermediate complexes with enzymatic activity have been encircled*

of tulips' under the electron microscope. The reaction of IgM or IgG antibody with antigen causes a conformational change in the Fc region of the antibody to reveal a binding site for C1q. C1q reacts with Fc via its globular heads but attachment by *two* critically spaced binding sites is needed for activation. The Fc regions of pentameric IgM are so spaced that one IgM molecule can activate C1q: in contrast, IgG is relatively inefficient because the chance of two randomly sited IgG molecules being the critical distance apart to activate C1q is relatively low. IgA, IgD and IgE do not activate the classical pathway and there are also differences in the ability of IgG subclasses to perform this role: IgG_1, IgG_3 and to a lesser extent IgG_2, but not IgG_4, can bind C1q.

Once C1q is bound by antibody, C1r and C1s are sequentially activated to generate enzyme activity for C4 and C2 (*Figure 4.4*), splitting both molecules into a and b fragments. The bimolecular complex $\overline{C4b2a}$ is the *classical pathway C3 convertase*. Other fragments released are C4a, C2b and a kinin-like peptide derived from C2. The C2a component of the C3 convertase rapidly decays and is the main limiting factor at this stage of the sequence.

$\overline{C4b2a}$ cleaves C3 into two fragments (*Figure 4.5*), one (C3a) possessing anaphylatoxic and chemotactic activity and one (C3b) which binds to the initiating immune complex and promotes many of the biological properties of complement.

The C4b2a3b complex so generated is an enzyme (C5 convertase) able to split C5 into a cell-bound fragment C5b and a minor fragment C5a, which also has chemotactic and anaphylatoxic properties. Once C5 has been cleaved, the remaining steps of the attack sequence are not enzymatic.

Alternative pathway activation

The central reaction in the alternative pathway, as in the classical one, is the activation of C3 (*Figure 4.6*). This pathway, however, generates a C3 convertase without the help of bound antibody, C1, C4 or C2. Instead, activation is induced by a range of substances, the most important being bacterial lipopolysaccharides. The alternative pathway is responsible for immediate defence against invading organisms, as it functions in the absence of preformed specific antibody.

The major proteins of the alternative pathway are properdin, factor B, factor D and C3 itself, together with the control proteins factor I (previously called C3b inactivator) and factor H (previously called β1H globulin). The pathway functions as a continuously cycling, positive-feedback loop in which two C3 convertases are formed (*Figure 4.6*). The initial or 'priming' convertase (C3Bb) is derived from native C3 and factor B. The effect of factor D is to split factor B and convert the complex to C3Bb. This 'priming' convertase is slowly formed even in the absence of activating agents, so continuously generating a low level of C3b which can then initiate formation of the second or 'amplification' C3 convertase, C3bBb. However, C3bBb rapidly becomes inactivated by spontaneous dissociation of the Bb subunit: properdin seems to stabilize the convertase by binding to it and retarding dissociation of Bb. Under appropriate circumstances, the resulting cell-bound complex C3bBbP is a stable and effective C3 convertase. The addition of another C3b molecule generates a properdin-stabilized amplification C5 convertase (C3b, Bb, C3b, P) which triggers activation of the attack sequence.

The functions of C3b and C3bBb are regulated by the control proteins H and I. H competes with factor B and the Bb fragment for binding to C3b, so limiting formation of the C3 convertase C3bBb, dissociating any formed C3bBb and increasing the susceptibility of C3b to cleavage by I.

The competition between H and factor B is influenced by the amounts of sialic acid and heparin present on the cell or particle surface; sialic acid promotes the binding of C3b to H rather than to factor B. Natural activators of the alternative pathway lack or possess only small amounts of sialic acid, thus favouring the binding of C3b to factor B and the formation of the C3 convertase C3bBb.

The fundamental difference between classical and alternative pathways is that, in the latter, C3b itself forms the essential component of the C3-splitting enzyme, enabling this pathway to amplify C3 activation, irrespective of how C3 cleavage is initially produced.

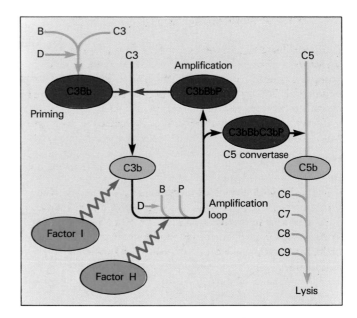

Figure 4.6 *Alternative pathway activation: the 'priming' convertase is continuously formed in small amounts. The resulting C3b itself participates in the 'amplification' convertase, generating more C3b. The pathway thus functions as a continuously cycling positive feedback loop: its effects are modulated by factor I and factor H at the points shown*

The 'attack' sequence

The attack sequence is thought to be the same irrespective of whether the C3 convertase is formed via the classical ($\overline{C4b2a}$) or alternative ($\overline{C3bBbP}$) pathways. Only the first step is enzymatic; this splits C5 into C5a and C5b. The remaining steps involve the sequential formation of a macromolecular complex comprising single molecules of C5b, C6, C7 and C8 and six molecules of C9. The $\overline{C567}$ complex can bind firmly to cell membranes, so localizing the subsequent lesion, but unbound $\overline{C567}$ loses its attachment site and forms a factor with chemotactic properties. Bound $\overline{C567}$ has a receptor site for C8 and its cofactor C9, the resulting complex inserting itself into the cell membrane, causing disruption of the lipid layer and resulting in ultrastructural 'holes' in the cell membrane.

Modulation of complement activation

Control systems regulate the results of complement activation; otherwise, once triggered, complement consumption would continue until the components were exhausted. The rapid decay of active sites and the action of specific inhibitors ensure that potentially harmful effects are confined to the initiating antigen without affecting host cells.

C1 inhibitor

This inhibitor combines with activated C1, but not native C1, to block its enzymatic action. It also inhibits plasmin, kallikrein and activated factors XI and XII of the clotting system. Absence of the inhibitor allows the unrestrained activity of C1 on C4 and C2 which are consumed to exhaustion.

Factor I

C3b is cleaved by I into two further fragments, C3c and C3d. When the inactivator splits cell- or complex-bound C3b, C3c is released but C3d remains attached, so preventing the unrestrained activity of the amplification loop of the alternative pathway; in the absence of I the amplification loop continuously cycles to exhaustion, causing a secondary deficiency of C3 (see below).

Factor H

The action of this protein is discussed above.

Biological effects of complement

Although the complete sequence of component activation is required for cell lysis, this is not necessarily the most important effect mediated by the system. Activation of C3 is the key step because C3b mediates a number of vital biological activities (*Table 4.1*).

Table 4.1 Biological properties of complement components

Component or fragment	Property
C1	Virus neutralization
C1q	Initiation of viral lysis
C2 kinin	Increased vascular permeability
C3a	Anaphylatoxin Chemotaxin
C3b	Immune adherence Opsonization Leucocyte mobilization from bone marrow
C4b	Immune adherence Initiation of viral lysis
C5a	Chemotaxin Anaphylatoxin
C5b67	Chemotaxin
C5-C9	Cell lysis

Immune adherence

Many cells, including macrophages, polymorphs, B lymphocytes and erythrocytes possess receptors for C3b. C3b-mediated immune adherence of certain cells to immune complexes may be an important prelude to phagocytosis or antigen presentation to B lymphocytes.

Opsonization

Immune complexes coated with C3b are ingested more readily by phagocytic cells than complexes lacking bound C3b. Since opsonic activity can be generated via the alternative pathway, this is an important means of defence against microorganisms in the nonimmune host.

Chemotaxins

Chemotaxins are substances that induce the directional migration of leucocytes along a concentration gradient of the agent. C3a, C5a and the C5b67 complex have chemotactic activity.

Anaphylatoxins

Both C3a and C5a have anaphylatoxic activity, although C5a is relatively weak.

Other biological activities

In vitro studies suggest that C1 and C4b can neutralize certain viruses coated with non-neutralizing antibodies, while C1q may bind directly to some oncornaviruses to induce complement-mediated lysis in the absence of antibody.

Laboratory assessment of complement activity

Three main groups of tests are available:
(1) Functional complement assays.
(2) Immunochemical measurement of individual components.
(3) Detection of complement breakdown products.

Collection of samples

Complement decays rapidly if stored inadequately, so all functional tests are subject to some risk of artefact. Ideally, sera should be tested fresh or stored frozen in suitably sized aliquots at −70°C. Refrozen sera are generally unsuitable.

Functional assays

Classical pathway function is assessed by the ability of complement to haemolyse erythrocytes coated with anti-red-cell antibodies. Screening assays (*Figure 4.7*) or more time-honoured tube assays are readily available: usually results are expressed in CH_{50} units, one unit being the volume of serum needed to lyse 50% of sensitized red cells under standard conditions.

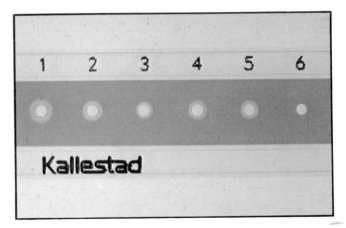

Figure 4.7 *Functional assay of classical pathway activity. Test serum is placed in wells cut into agarose gel containing antibody-sensitized sheep erythrocytes. If all complement components are present in sufficient quantities, a radial zone of lysis is produced, the ring diameter being proportional to the amount of functional complement present. In the slide shown, doubling dilutions of a complement standard have been added to wells 1 to 3 and neat test sera to wells 4 to 6. The absence of lysis around well 6 is very suggestive of an inherited complement deficiency*

Haemolytic assays also can assess alternative pathway and individual component activities. Although such functional tests are highly specific, they are expensive, time-consuming and seldom necessary in clinical practice other than in the detection of genetic defects (see p. 43).

Immunochemical assays

The most widely available tests are immunochemical measurements of certain components using specific antisera. Normal levels may be found even when functional activity has decayed through poor storage. However, under rare circumstances some components lack functional activity and yet are detectable in significant amounts by immunochemical methods.

Complement breakdown products

Activation products resulting from *in vivo* complement cleavage can be distinguished from the native components by differences in their electrophoretic charge. Unfortunately, clotting generates *in vitro* artefacts although these can be avoided largely by taking blood into EDTA.

Clinical interpretation of changes in complement

Blood levels of complement components at any time are the net result of complement synthesis versus utilization and catabolism. Thus, high levels may be due to increased production or to reduced utilization and catabolism and conversely, low levels could reflect impaired synthesis or increased consumption and catabolism. Apparently normal levels can occur if heightened synthesis is balanced by hypercatabolism. To some extent, such difficulties in interpretation are overcome by serial measurements.

Raised complement levels

Many components behave as acute phase reactants: total haemolytic activity, and levels of individual proteins are raised (*Table 4.2*) during a variety of acute inflammatory conditions. Complement measurement in such circumstances is of limited value, other than as a parameter of the effect of treatment.

Table 4.2 Interpretation of changes in serum complement

Change in complement component				Implied pattern of activation
CH$_{50}$	C4	C3	Factor B	
↓	↓	↓	N	Classical pathway
↓	N	↓	↓	Alternative pathway
↓	↓	↓	↓	Classical and alternative pathway
↑	↑	↑	↑	Acute phase response

Low complement levels

Low or absent complement activity provides evidence of:
(1) Immunologically mediated complement consumption via either the classical or alternative pathways.
(2) Impaired complement synthesis.
(3) Inherited primary deficiencies of complement components or their inhibitors.

General principles

To understand the changes in serum complement in disease, it is useful to consider the complement components in three groups (*Figure 4.8*): early components of the classical pathway (C1qrs, C4 and C2); early components of the alternative pathway (properdin, factor B and factor D); late components common to both pathways (C3 to C9 inclusive).

When the classical pathway is activated, there is utilization of C1 to C9 with relative sparing of alternative pathway proteins. This pattern is most commonly found in soluble immune complex diseases, such as SLE. If the alternative pathway is principally involved, one would expect a fall in the alternative pathway and attack sequence component levels with sparing of early classical pathway proteins. Such a pattern is seen in severe gram-negative bacteraemia and endotoxic shock. However, when C3b is generated via classical pathway activity, there is the potential for subsequent activation of the alternative

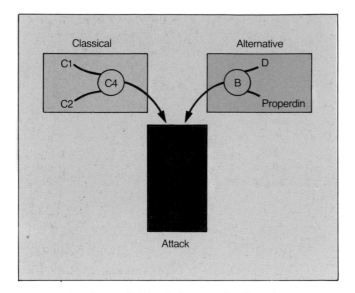

Figure 4.8 *Principles underlying the interpretation of complement profiles. It is useful to consider proteins of the complement system in three groups, of which C4, C3 and factor B are representative and most readily measured*

pathway by the feedback loop. Levels of alternative pathway components therefore must be interpreted with this possibility in mind.

In practice (*Table 4.2*), low C4 and C3 but normal factor B levels suggest that activation of the classical pathway alone has occurred; if C4, C3 and factor B levels are low, the alternative pathway probably is also activated, either via the feedback loop or by independent activation. Normal C4 levels with reduced C3 and factor B provide evidence for activation of the alternative pathway alone.

Complement levels in immune complex diseases

Systemic lupus erythematosus

The pattern of complement activation in SLE varies with the type of organ involvement. Patients with renal disease show consumption and glomerular deposition of early classical pathway components, leading to low serum C4

and C3 levels which return to normal during clinical remission. Serial observations indicate that complement levels, particularly C4, fall before other features of relapse become apparent; C4 and C3 are thus useful parameters of the effectiveness of treatment and early indicators of deterioration. In addition, low serum levels and glomerular deposition of factor B indicates some activation of the alternative pathway.

In SLE without renal involvement, serum complement may be normal or alternatively a low C4 is found. Cerebrospinal fluid complement levels are an unreliable diagnostic tool in patients with cerebral lupus.

Rheumatoid arithritis

In most patients, complement levels are either normal or raised as part of the acute phase response. Low serum levels, however, may be found in strongly seropositive patients with associated vasculitis. Synovial fluid complement may be depressed in active rheumatoid arthritis because of complement consumption by immune complexes within the synovial space.

Cryoglobulinaemia

In mixed cryoglobulinaemia, the complexes activate and deplete the early classical pathway components C1q, C4 and C2.

Complement levels in renal disease

Complement levels are diagnostically helpful in patients with glomerulonephritis. Immune complex nephritis, such as SLE, cryoglobulin nephropathy, serum sickness and malaria, is accompanied by classical pathway activation and low levels of C4 and C3. In poststreptococcal glomerulonephritis, C4 levels are only mildly and variably depressed in early stages of the disease but soon return to normal; however, C3 levels show a marked lowering with a more gradual return to normal, in uncomplicated cases, over 8 to 12 weeks. This contrasts with mesangiocapillary glomerulonephritis in which profoundly depressed C3 levels persist despite normal C1, C4 and C2 concentrations.

Some patients have a serum factor, termed C3 nephritic factor (C3 NeF), which induces C3 activation via the alternative pathway. C3 NeF has also been found in most children with partial lipodystrophy even in the absence of overt renal disease. It is a polyclonal IgG autoantibody which binds to the alternative pathway convertase C3bBb to create a stable complex which is resistant to dissociation by factor H: as a result, C3 and factor B consumption are increased. The presence of C3 NeF is not related to the clinical state of the patient, but helps to differentiate between relatively benign, self-limiting, acute poststreptococcal glomerulonephritis and the more serious mesangiocapillary glomerulonephritis.

In many other forms of renal disease, such as minimal change disease, Goodpasture's syndrome, IgA nephropathy, Henoch–Schönlein disease, pyelonephritis, obstructive nephropathy and most forms of congenital renal disease, serum complement levels are of little diagnostic value.

Complement levels in liver disease

In the early stages of acute hepatitis B, C4 and C3 levels are often low, particularly in those cases with urticaria and arthritis. As symptoms subside and antibody titres rise, complement levels return to normal, suggesting that many of the clinical features are due to immune complex deposition. In some cases progressing to acute hepatic necrosis, persistently low C4 and C3 levels reflect impaired hepatic synthesis of these components with continued complement consumption. While changes in serum complement components have been recorded in cases of chronic liver disease, they are not of established diagnostic value.

Complement levels in infectious disease

The inflammatory response may include an acute phase rise in complement components: alternatively, low levels may reflect classical pathway activation by circulating immune complexes of antibody and microorganisms, or alternative pathway activation by bacterial lipopolysaccharide. For example, gram-negative bacteraemia is accompanied typically by the features of alternative pathway activation (*Table 4.2*), while subacute bacterial endocarditis, nephritis associated with infected ventriculoatrial shunts, and acute malaria show low levels of C1, C4 and C3.

Inherited defects in complement

In humans, inherited deficiencies of components of the complement system are associated with four characteristic clinical syndromes (*Figure 4.9*):

(1) An increased susceptibility to recurrent bacterial infections in patients with C3 deficiency (occurring as a primary defect or secondary to deficiency of either factor I or factor H) or properdin deficiency.

(2) An increased incidence of immune complex disorders or lupus-like syndromes associated with early classical pathway component deficiencies.

(3) An increased susceptibility to recurrent or chronic Neisseria infections in patients with genetic defects of one of the 'attack' sequence proteins.

(4) Hereditary angioedema in patients with genetic deficiency of C1 inhibitor.

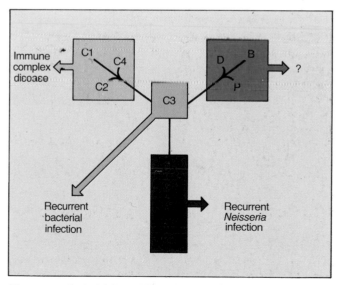

Figure 4.9 *Inherited defects in complement: characteristic clinical syndromes are associated with deficiencies of certain groups of components*

Inherited defects are rare but highlight the importance of an intact complement system. The defect (with the exception of C1 inhibitor deficiency) usually results in complete absence of haemolytic activity and the missing protein can be identified by functional and immunochemical tests. In some cases, a nonfunctioning but immunochemically detectable protein is present.

Primary C3 deficiency

Affected individuals typically present with recurrent infections by pyogenic bacteria, usually pneumonia, septicaemia, otitis media and bacterial meningitis. The patients lack C3, while first-degree relatives heterozygous for the abnormal gene have no undue susceptibility to infection despite their half-normal C3 levels. Most complement-mediated functions such as haemolytic activity, opsonization of endotoxin, bactericidal activity and leucocyte mobilization are markedly depressed or absent, illustrating the vital role of C3. In contrast, antibody production is normal.

Factor I deficiency

Only five patients with inherited deficiency of factor I have been described. The first patient had a lifelong history of severe bacterial infections including septicaemia, pneumonia, meningitis, sinusitis and otitis media; the other patients also had several episodes of pyogenic infection.

In the absence of factor I, C3b causes continued overaction and exhaustion of the alternative pathway via the amplification loop. Thus patients had increased C3 turnover with low serum levels of C3 and factor B, but normal C1, C4 and C2 concentrations. These defects were reversible by plasma infusion and by replacement of purified factor I.

Factor H deficiency

The first report of H deficiency was that of a Pakistani infant who presented with the haemolytic–uraemic syndrome. He was found to have a low serum C3 level which persisted despite clinical improvement. The child had a very low level of H, with evidence of continued alternative pathway activation, despite a normal level of I. An asymptomatic 3-year-old brother had an identical abnormality.

Defects of early classical pathway components

Inherited deficiencies of each of these proteins show a similar clinical picture: most patients with C1q, C1r, C1s, C4 or C2 deficiency have presented with lupus-like syndromes of malar flush, arthralgia, glomerulonephritis, recurrent fever, or chronic vasculitis, and sometimes with recurrent pyogenic infection. Many of the patients, however, lack lupus erythematosus cells, antinuclear or anti-ds DNA antibodies.

The defect is usually inherited as an autosomal recessive trait, affected subjects being homozygous for the abnormal gene. Heterozygotes can be detected by their half-normal functional or immunochemical serum concentrations of the protein. Evidence in one case of C1q deficiency suggested that the defect resulted from an abnormal gene producing a nonfunctional but antigenically cross-reactive C1q molecule.

With the exception of hereditary angioedema, C2 deficiency is the commonest complement deficiency, the frequency of the abnormal gene being estimated at 1%. Among reported C2-deficient subjects, between 30% and 40% have been clinically healthy.

Development of immune complex disease

The intriguing question is why patients with deficiencies of this type apparently develop immune complex diseases. There seem to be four possibilities. First, the association may be a detection artefact because complement levels are measured most frequently in patients with immune complex diseases and therefore complement deficiencies also will be found most frequently in this group. Second, the complement deficiency itself may not be related causally to the immune complex disorder but may be a marker for a closely linked genetic locus which determines the disease. This argument particularly applies to C2 or C4 deficiency, where linkage of the C4 and C2 genes to the major histocompatibility complex is established. However, genes controlling the other early pathways components (C1q, C1r and C1s) do not show HLA linkage. The third possibility is that deficiency of any protein needed to form the classical pathway C3 convertase compromises the ability of the host to eliminate antigens, particularly viruses, so leading to immune complex disease. There is some evidence that lupus-like syndromes in animals and humans may be due to persistent viral infection. Finally, deficiency of an early component of the classical pathway may cause antigen–antibody complexes to precipitate at or near their site of formation and lead to immunologically mediated inflammation. The classical complement pathway has an important role in keeping immune complexes soluble long enough for their safe removal by the mononuclear phagocyte system.

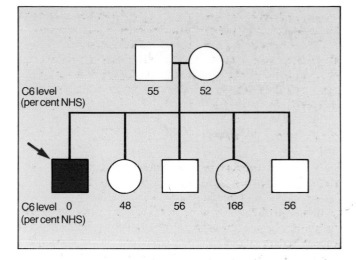

Figure 4.10 *C6 levels in a C6-deficient patient (arrowed) and his family. Values are expressed as a percentage of a normal human serum (NHS). Individuals with proposed homozygous C6 deficiency are shown in red, and those with proposed heterozygous C6 deficiency in yellow*

Deficiencies of 'attack' sequence components

There is a striking association between deficiencies of C5, C6, C7 or C8 and recurrent Neisseria infection. Affected individuals have presented with recurrent gonococcal infection, particularly septicaemia and arthritis, or recurrent meningococcal meningitis. The true frequency of the defect is difficult to determine: a high index of clinical suspicion is essential since episodes of meningitis may be many years apart. Despite high serum titres of complement-fixing antibody to meningococci, bactericidal activity is absent until restored by the addition of fresh complement (*Table 4.3*), suggesting that complement-mediated lysis is a

vital defence against Neisseria infection. Deficiencies of C5 to C8 appear to be inherited as autosomal recessive traits (*Figure 4.10*).

Deficiency of C9 has been reported in several patients, often of Russian–Jewish descent. No patient has had any history of recurrent or unusual infection or autoimmune disease, which is in keeping with the experimental observation that C1 to C8 can induce slow lytic activity even in the absence of C9.

Table 4.3 Antimeningococcal antibody activity in a patient with C6 deficiency

		Antibody activity	
		Bactericidal antibody titre	
Days following onset of symptoms	Complement-fixing antibody titre	Patient's serum alone	Patient's serum plus fresh complement
+2	1/32	<1/2	1/16
+14	1/128	<1/2	1/128

Deficiencies of alternative pathway components

There have been no reported cases of inherited deficiency of factor B or factor D. However, the importance of the alternative pathway is suggested by the relatively low incidence of severe bacterial infection in patients who cannot form the classical pathway C3 convertase because of deficiencies of C1, C4 or C2.

C1 inhibitor deficiency

C1 inhibitor deficiency is the commonest inherited deficiency within the complement system and gives rise to the condition of hereditary angioneurotic oedema (HANE). This protein inhibits activated proteins of several systems including plasmin and kallikrein as well as C1. In its absence, these systems are subject to low-grade continuous activation, their combined effects exhausting any limited supplies of the inhibitor and allowing C1 to act on C4 and C2 to generate the C2 kinin-like peptide and some C3a anaphylatoxin.

The defect is inherited as an autosomal dominant trait. This is one of the few situations where the heterozygote exhibits the disease and highlights the critical need for a

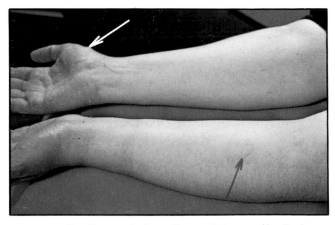

Figure 4.11 *Hereditary angioedema. Characteristic areas of localized oedema are present on the anterolateral aspect of the left forearm and the right thenar eminence (arrowed)*

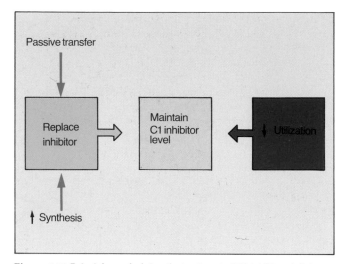

Figure 4.12 *Principles underlying the treatment of C1 inhibitor deficiency*

normal level of inhibitor. Acquired and spontaneous, nonfamilial forms have been described.

Patients suffer from recurrent attacks of peripheral, laryngeal or intestinal oedema. Localized oedema (*Figure 4.11*) of the limbs, face and trunk is neither painful nor itchy. Sometimes, however, oedema occurs in the intestinal tract, causing severe abdominal pain and vomiting when the jejunum is involved or watery diarrhoea if the colon is affected. Laryngeal oedema may be fatal because of airways obstruction. The attacks last 2–3 days and then subside spontaneously. Although often unheralded, episodes may occur after trauma, menstruation, stress or intercurrent infection. Attacks of angioedema are infrequent in early childhood; exacerbations occur during adolescence but tend to subside beyond the age of 60 years.

The diagnosis rests on finding low levels of C1 inhibitor. In active disease, uninhibited C1 cleaves C4 and C2, causing increased turnover and low levels. Although C3 turnover is slightly increased, serum levels are usually normal. A low serum C4 and normal C3 thus provide a useful screening test for this condition. Two forms of the disease seem to exist: in the common form (85%) no C1 inhibitor is found but in the rarer type (15%) a functionally defective protein is synthesized. Thus, in this latter group,

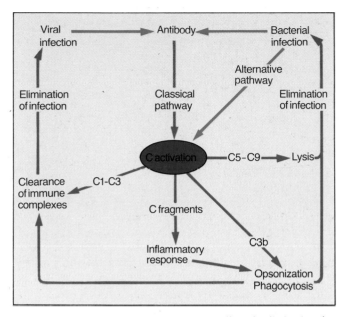

Figure 4.13 *Mechanisms by which complement effects the elimination of invading microorganisms. The dominant role of certain components is highlighted by the study of inherited deficiencies of complement (see text)*

serum levels of the inhibitor. Treatment with testosterone ethanate (Danazol) has been very effective in stimulating C1 inhibitor synthesis. εAminocaproic acid (EACA) and its analogue, tranexamic acid, are also effective prophylactic agents; they probably function by restricting activation of the various other enzymes with which C1 inhibitor reacts, so minimizing its consumption.

47

Conclusion

The inferences which can be drawn (*Figure 4.13*) from a study of inherited defects of complement components are that the early classical pathway is relatively unimportant in defence against bacterial infection but promotes the elimination of immune complexes, particularly those involving viruses. In contrast, the alternative complement pathway and C3 are very important in resistance to bacterial infection while the 'attack' sequence seems necessary for efficient elimination of Neisseria organisms.

Further reading

AGNELLO, V. (1978) Complement deficiency states. *Medicine (Baltimore)*, **57**, 1–23

LACHMANN, P. J. and ROSEN, F. S. (1978) Genetic defects of complement in man. *Springer Seminars in Immunopathology*, **1**, 339–353

SCHIFFERLI, J. A. and PETERS, D. K. (1983) Complement, the immune-complex lattice, and the pathophysiology of complement-deficiency syndromes. *Lancet*, **2**, 957–959

THOMPSON, R. A. (1983) Complement. In *Immunology in Medicine*, 2nd edn, pp. 95–119 (E. J. Holborow and W. G. Reeves, eds). Academic Press, London

there may be normal serum levels of an immunochemically cross-reacting but nonfunctioning inhibitor. In the patient with angioedema, a low C4 level but a normal immunochemical C1 inhibitor concentration indicates the need for a functional assay.

Symptoms normally fail to respond to antihistamines and respond poorly, if at all, to steroids. An acute attack can be treated (*Figure 4.12*) by infusion of fresh plasma to increase

5 Immune complexes and disease

Complexes of antigen and antibody are probably formed each time we make a humoral immune response to antigen challenge. This process may exert a significant regulatory effect on the immune system but rarely leads to tissue damage. Paradoxically, however, tissue deposition of circulating immune complexes is believed to contribute to the features of many diseases. This chapter considers why immune complexes may be organ-damaging in some individuals but harmless or even beneficial in others.

Principles of the antigen–antibody reaction

The classical 'precipitin reaction' illustrates the important features of antigen–antibody interaction. If gradually increasing amounts of an antigen are added to a series of tubes containing a fixed amount of specific antibody (*Figure 5.1a*), precipitates will appear in some tubes after incubation, reaching a maximum at a certain antigen concentration: addition of further antigen will dissolve the precipitate. Thus, the typical precipitin curve (*Figure 5.1b*), in which the weight of the precipitate is plotted against the amount of antigen added, shows a gradual increase in precipitate followed by a fall as more antigen is added. The point at which the sites of both antigen and antibody are saturated is called the equivalence point of the curve.

These observations and the clinical relevance of the antigen–antibody ratio are best explained by the lattice hypothesis (*Figure 5.2*). Most antigens have many antigenic determinants (that is, multivalent antigens), while antibodies possess at least two combining sites. At equivalence, antigen molecules are cross-linked by antibody to form a large, precipitable lattice. When further antigen is added, the antibody-combining sites in the Fab regions are blocked and cannot fully cross-link, so preventing precipitation but allowing the formation of small soluble complexes instead. Soluble complexes may also be formed in antibody excess (*Figure 5.2*), but it follows that cross-linkage and hence precipitation cannot occur with those antigens consisting of a single antigenic determinant.

Biological effects of immune complexes

The physiological effects of immune complexes depend upon the properties of the antigen and antibody components and on their ability to bind to various cellular and humoral receptors (*Figure 5.3*).

Complement activation

Immune complexes activate the complement system, mainly via the classical pathway, and generate several important biological effects (see Chapter 4). The anaphylatoxic and chemotactic properties of certain fragments promote the migration of phagocytic and other cells into the area of immune complex deposition. Recognition of complex-bound C3b by receptors on macrophages, polymorphs and B lymphocytes may be important in localizing and retaining these cells before phagocytosis of the complexes or before modulation of the immune response. Immune complexes coated with C3b are more readily ingested by phagocytic cells than complexes lacking bound

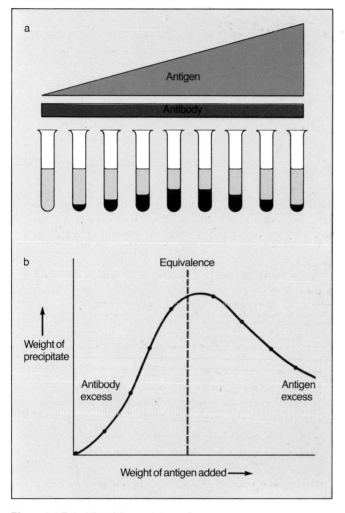

Figure 5.1 *Principles of the precipitin reaction between a single antigen and a specific antiserum. See text for explanation*

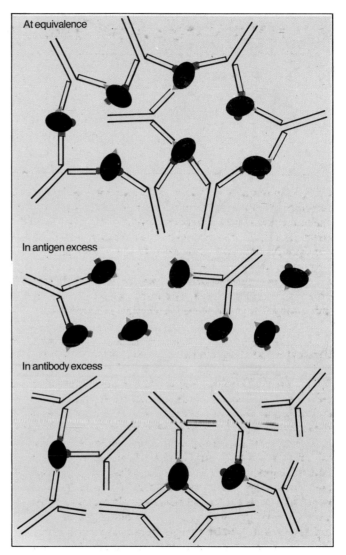

Figure 5.2 *Diagrammatic representation of immune complexes formed at equivalence, in extreme antigen excess and in extreme antibody excess*

C3b. Lysis of invading microorganisms occurs through the action of the components of the complement attack sequence (C3 to C9) when an immune complex is formed between a cell-surface antigen and a complement-activating antibody.

However, there is experimental evidence that the damaging inflammatory response associated with immune complex deposition may be mediated partly via the activation of complement (see below).

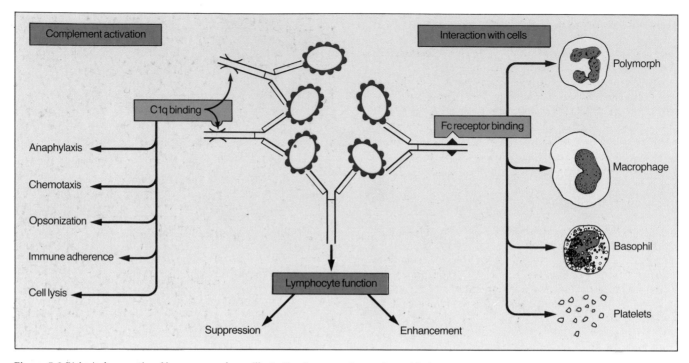

Figure 5.3 *Biological properties of immune complexes, illustrating important interactions with the complement system, lymphocytes and other cells*

Interaction with cells

Immune complexes interact with receptors present on the surfaces of various cells (*Figure 5.3*).

Neutrophils and mononuclear phagocytes

These cells possess receptors for the Fc region of IgG. Attachment of antibody-coated antigens to Fc receptors is followed by phagocytosis, with a concomitant release of proteolytic enzymes, lysozyme and basic peptides capable of increasing vascular permeability, stimulating mast cells and indirectly activating the clotting system. Most of the immune complexes appearing in the circulation are normally cleared by cells of the mononuclear phagocyte system (MPS).

Mast cells and basophils

These cells can bind IgE antibody (and probably some IgG subclass antibody). Binding of cell-fixed antibody to a multivalent antigen, or the exposure of these cells to complement fragments C3a and C5a, is followed by the release of mediators such as histamine and leukotrienes.

Platelets

Human platelets have receptors for the Fc region of IgG. Thus immune complexes containing IgG cause platelet aggregation and the release of vasoactive proteins and procoagulant factors.

Effects of complexes on lymphocyte function

Immune complexes may, in the appropriate circumstances, suppress or enhance immune function.

Suppression of immune responses is well recognized: a simple explanation is that the antigen component is masked by antibody and hence not recognized by antigen-specific cell receptors. Other additional mechanisms are possible: complexes may block antigen receptors on either B lymphocytes or helper T cells, inhibit the cooperative interactions between these and other cells, or suppress plasma cells directly.

Immune complexes may alternatively augment the immune response. Complexes, especially those in antigen excess, are reported to be more immunogenic than free antigens, both for primary and secondary antibody responses. This enhancement has been attributed variously to the improved processing of antigen by macrophages, to increased binding of complexed antigen by lymphocytes and to better cooperation between B and T lymphocytes.

Whether complexes suppress or enhance the immune response is critically dependent upon such factors as the antigen–antibody ratio and the class and affinity of antibody.

Fate of immune complexes

A study of immune complex diseases poses two major questions: how are circulating immune complexes normally removed from the body, and why do these clearance mechanisms fail and immune complexes persist in some individuals? Partial answers to these questions are provided by experimental models in which deposition of immune complexes is triggered by single or repeated exposure to antigen.

Experimental models

Acute ('one-shot') serum sickness

A single intravenous injection of a foreign antigen into rabbits causes an illness, 10–12 days later, characterized by

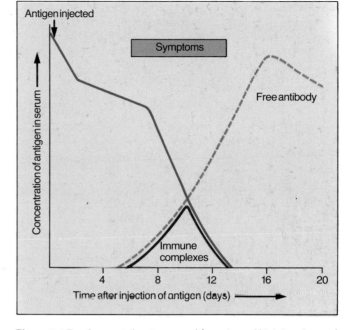

51

Figure 5.4 *Development of acute serum sickness in a rabbit injected intravenously with a single dose of antigen. The onset of symptoms and proteinuria coincides with the appearance of immune complexes in the circulation*

arthritis, glomerulonephritis and arteritis. Following injection, the antigen disappears from the circulation in three stages (*Figure 5.4*): an initial phase, lasting 1–2 days, during which the antigen becomes equilibrated between intravascular and extravascular spaces; a second phase representing normal catabolism of the antigen, followed by a final phase of rapid immune elimination. During this latter phase, antigen-antibody complexes are detectable in the circulation at the same time that damage is produced in the glomeruli, joints and blood vessels of the experimental animal. Immunofluorescent examination of the lesions shows deposition of antigen, antibody and complement along the glomerular basement membrane and in blood vessel walls. In most instances, this symptomatic phase is short-lived and rapidly subsides, with complete healing, as complexes are cleared by the MPS. Elimination of antigen is accompanied by the appearance of free antibodies in the circulation.

Chronic experimental immune complex disease

In the classic chronic serum sickness model, rabbits are given daily intravenous injections of a low dose of foreign antigen. This process may, after 2–3 months, result in chronic, progressive glomerulonephritis in some animals. The lesions do not depend on the characteristics of the antigen but the amount of antigen given is critical. The key requirement is to produce a state of antigen excess after each injection, thus saturating free antibody and generating daily infusions of immune complexes. Significantly, using this experimental protocol, some animals neither produce an antibody response nor develop glomerulonephritis (*Figure 5.5a*), while rabbits showing very poor antibody production require longer periods of repeated injections before renal damage occurs. Thus, some degree of humoral immune response seems necessary to provoke tissue injury. Conversely, chronic glomerulonephritis is difficult to induce in animals making a strong immune response (*Figure 5.5b*), as further antigen administration only results in rapid elimination of antigen. In order to generate chronic immune complex disease the animal must make just enough antibody to remain in the zone of antigen excess (*Figure 5.5c*).

Using a different protocol, in which the daily antigen dose is adjusted to ensure slight antigen excess even in good antibody formers (*Figure 5.5d*), it is possible to induce chronic serum sickness in virtually every rabbit. When free antibodies appear in the circulation, the injection of further low amounts of antigen causes only the formation of large, insoluble complexes which are rapidly cleared by the MPS and by mesangial cells in the kidney. However, increasing the antigen load will, after a variable time, lead to the formation of circulating complexes in antigen excess which are small enough to be deposited in the glomerular capillary wall and provoke a progressive glomeru-lonephritis.

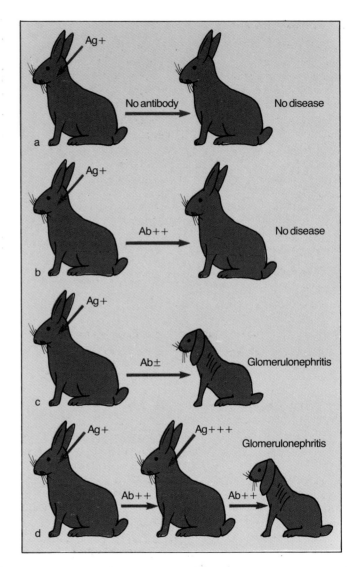

Figure 5.5 *Chronic experimental immune complex disease: the development of lesions after daily intravenous injections of antigen is dependent on the quality of antibody produced by the rabbit. Animals producing (a) no antibody or (b) strong-affinity antibody (Ab+ +) remain well but animals forming low-affinity antibody (Ab±) develop chronic glomerulonephritis (c). If the daily antigen load is increased (Ag+ to Ag+ + +) it is possible to induce serum sickness even in good antibody producers (d)*

The Arthus reaction

In the Arthus reaction, first described in 1903, local, immune-complex-mediated inflammation is induced by injection of antigen into the skin of a previously immunized animal producing a high circulating antibody titre. A haemorrhagic, oedematous reaction develops in the skin over 4–8 hours and persists for 12–24 hours. Because the complexes form locally in the tissue, they can occur at equivalence as well as in antigen excess. At one time, when antitoxin or antibacterial sera frequently were administered to provide passive immunity, the Arthus reaction was relatively common. It may still occur in any situation in which antibodies react locally with free or tissue-bound antigens, and this mechanism may be operative in the pathogenesis of many conditions, including extrinsic allergic alveolitis, coeliac disease and certain forms of glomerulonephritis.

Normal clearance of immune complexes

The MPS is the major protective mechanism against tissue deposition of circulating immune complexes. Phagocytic cells have Fc receptors, and the binding of these to IgG enhances the clearance of complexes. The fate of immune complexes depends principally upon their size. Very large, insoluble complexes are removed rapidly from the circulation by the MPS, particularly by the Kupffer cells of the liver. Very small, soluble complexes do not localize in tissues or cause damage. Biologically active complexes seem to be of intermediate size: they are cleared poorly from the circulation and can fix to vessel walls, renal glomeruli or the choroid plexus. The exact location of complexes within these particular tissues is also size-dependent. For example, in the glomerulus, two main patterns of immune complex deposition are seen. First, deposits may be present on the epithelial side of the glomerular basement membrane: it is thought that they are either formed locally or represent small immune complexes which have undergone progressive aggregation during passage through the basement membrane. Second, deposits may occur mainly in the mesangium and, to a lesser extent, between the endothelium and the basement

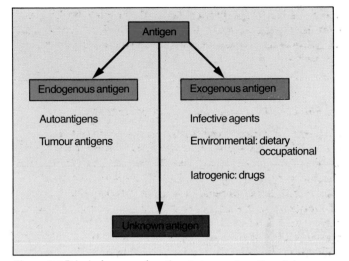

Figure 5.6 *Principal sources of continued exposure to antigen in humans*

membrane: these deposits may be relatively large complexes unable to penetrate the basement membrane.

Persistent generation of immune complexes

Immune complex formation would be expected to persist or recur, if there is either continued exposure to the antigen or a failure by the host to deal with formed complexes.

Causes of continued exposure to antigen

By analogy with the rabbit model of serum sickness, a chronic state of antigen excess should also induce immune complex disease in man (*Figure 5.6*).

There is some evidence that exposure to environmental antigens, particularly those of dietary origin, may be followed by the appearance of circulating complexes, but the role of these complexes in causing tissue damage is debatable.

The commonest recognized source of antigen is infection (*Table 5.1*). Immune complexes are difficult to detect in acute infection, where circulation time is short, but are frequently found in chronic viral or parasitic infection where persistent replication of the microorganism occurs in

Table 5.1 Immune complex diseases in man

Antigen[a]	Associated disease[b]	Antigen[a]	Associated disease[b]
(1) Exogenous antigens		Drugs	
Viruses		Probenecid	Drug-induced nephropathy
Hepatitis B	Hepatitis B	Penicillamine	
	Polyarteritis nodosa	Mercury	
	Mixed essential cryoglobulinaemia	Gold	
Cytomegalovirus	Glomerulonephritis	Heroin	
Epstein-Barr virus	Infectious mononucleosis	Foreign serum	Serum sickness
	Burkitt's lymphoma	Dietary antigens	
	Nasopharyngeal carcinoma	Gluten	Coeliac disease
Measles	Subacute sclerosing panencephalitis	Others	Asthma/eczema
Oncornavirus	Leukaemia	**(2) Endogenous antigens**	
	Lymphoma	Autoantigens	
Dengue	Dengue haemorrhagic fever	Nuclear products	SLE
Bacteria			Scleroderma
Streptococcus	Poststreptococcal glomerulonephritis	Thyroglobulin	Hashimoto's disease
Streptococcus viridans	Bacterial endocarditis	Renal tubular antigen	Membranous nephropathy
Staphylococcus	Shunt nephritis		Renal vein thrombosis
Mycobacterium leprae	Lepromatous leprosy		Sickle cell anaemia
Treponema pallidum	Syphilis	Carcinoembryonic antigen	Carcinoma
Parasites		IgG	Rheumatoid arthritis
Plasmodium malariae	Quartan malarial nephropathy		Cryoglobulinaemia
Schistosoma mansoni	Schistosoma glomerulonephritis	Tumour antigens	
Toxoplasma gondii	Toxoplasma glomerulonephritis	Tumour-specific antigens	Neoplasia

[a]In other disorders with features suggestive of immune complex deposition no specific antigen has been incriminated
[b]While immune complexes have been detected in these conditions, other mechanisms may also contribute to the pathogenesis of the tissue lesions

spite of a host response. Although many infections are associated with tissue changes suggestive of immune complex deposits, recovery of the implicated antigen from the lesion has been achieved in only a minority of cases.

Failure to eliminate immune complexes

Immune complexes will persist if there is a failure of primary mechanisms for disposal of these complexes:

failure might be induced by the properties of the antigen, the nature of the antibody response or a dysfunction of complement or the MPS (*Figure 5.7*).

Properties of the antigen

Cross-linkage of antigen molecules by antibody will be limited if the antigen possesses few determinants. Impaired lattice formation is associated with poor clearance of

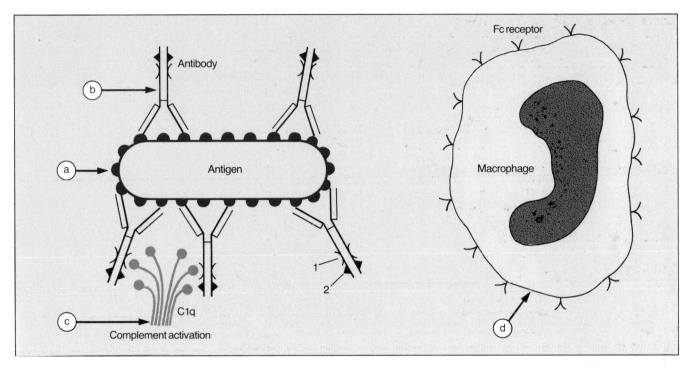

Figure 5.7 *Failure to clear circulating immune complexes can result from properties possessed by the antigen (a), an inadequate antibody response (b), impaired complement activation (c) or dysfunction of the MPS (d). Determinants are present in the Fc region of IgG capable of binding to C1q (1) or to Fc receptors on cell membranes (2)*

complexes by phagocytes. In some circumstances, a massive antigen load will ensure antigen excess in spite of reasonable amounts of circulating antibody: this may occur in drug hypersensitivity or infection.

Antibody response

In the experimental model of immune complex disease, relatively few animals develop chronic glomerulonephritis in spite of repeated, low-dose antigen exposure. Affected animals, however, produce mainly nonprecipitating anti-bodies to the injected antigen. This may be because the antibody binds weakly to the antigen, that is, it is of low affinity. Low-affinity antibody is poor at antigen elimina-tion, and mouse strains inbred to produce low-affinity

antibody to certain viruses are very susceptible to immune complex disease when specifically exposed to these infections in the neonatal period. By analogy, it is possible that individuals suffering from immune complex diseases are those who produce low-affinity antibody to the relevant antigen.

Clearance of immune complexes may be impaired also if the MPS lacks receptors for the class or subclass of the antibody component.

Complement defects

The complement system has an important role in solubiliz-ing immune complexes. There is evidence that deficiencies of some complement components are associated with immune complex disorders. Many patients with inherited deficiencies of the early classical pathway proteins (C1q, C1r, C1s, C4 or C2) present with lupus-like syndromes of malar flush, arthralgia, glomerulonephritis or vasculitis.

Phagocyte dysfunction

It appears, from experimental evidence, that the MPS is responsible for the clearance of passively administered, large immune complexes. If the phagocytic capacity of this system is saturated, immune complex retention in the circulation and subsequent tissue deposition is correspondingly increased. Recent studies have shown a markedly impaired clearance of injected preformed immune complexes in patients with untreated SLE. While the precise reason for this dysfunction is not known, saturation of the Fc receptors on tissue macrophages by deposited complexes may be responsible.

Pathological effects of immune complex deposition

There are two major clinical considerations: first, what factors influence the apparently preferential deposition of immune complexes in certain organs, and second, what mechanisms are then responsible for the tissue injury?

Tissue factors influencing immune complex deposition

Certain organs, such as the glomerulus, choroid plexus, skin, synovium and blood vessels, are repeatedly involved as sites of immune complex injury. One possible explanation is that some of these tissues contain potential receptors for components of the immune complex (*Table 5.2*).

Human glomerular epithelial cells possess receptors which recognize the activated C3 component of complement. Surprisingly, such receptors have been described only in human glomeruli. The apparent absence of the receptor from the glomeruli of rabbits, where the capacity to develop experimental immune complex disease is well established, raises some doubts about the *in vivo* relevance of the receptor to human disease and questions the evolutionary benefit to healthy individuals of possessing such a structure.

Clinical and experimental observations suggest that receptors for the Fc portion of IgG also occur in human choroid plexus, renal interstitium and placenta where they may play some role in the tissue injury characteristic of the cerebral and renal features of SLE or pre-eclamptic toxaemia, respectively.

The antigen may also influence the site of complex deposition. There is some evidence that DNA possesses unique properties which allow it to adhere to glomerular basement membrane: this may explain partly the frequency of renal involvement in SLE.

Mechanisms of tissue injury

Antigen–antibody complexes localized in and around the walls of blood vessels initiate a damaging inflammatory response mediated through the activation of complement and the influx and participation of phagocytic cells (*Figure 5.8*).

Complement activation can occur if the antibody is mainly IgM or IgG and the release of chemotactic factors encourages the migration of polymorphs and macrophages into the area. The binding of complexes to cell membranes, via the Fc and C3b receptors, facilitates phagocytosis of complexes and the discharge of lysosomal enzymes, including tissue-damaging proteases, collagenases and elastases. Enzyme release is partly a passive process following cell death and partly an active selective process of

Table 5.2 Possible tissue receptors detecting components of immune complexes

Tissue	Receptor
Renal glomerulus	C3b
Renal tubular basement membrane	Fc
Choroid plexus	Fc
Placenta	Fc

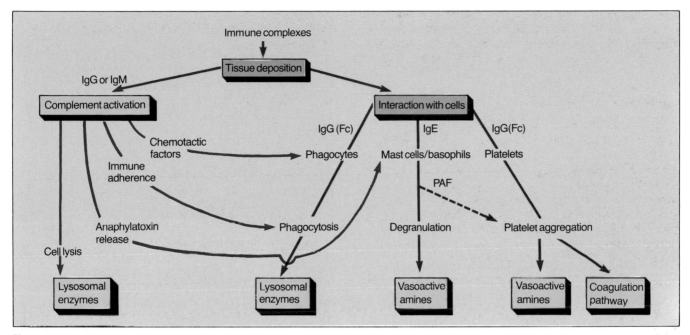

Figure 5.8 *Simplified view of the major pathways by which immune complex deposition may produce tissue damage (PAF=platelet aggregating factor)*

'reverse endocytosis' triggered by the interaction of complexes with cell-surface receptors.

The arteritis seen in the rabbit model of acute serum sickness can be inhibited by experimental depletion of either polymorphs or complement before the 'single shot' of antigen. However, complement and polymorph depletion does not arrest the development of glomerular injury, indicating that other processes must be involved.

Vasoactive amines released from platelets, mast cells and basophils cause increased vascular permeability and may enhance the deposition of immune complexes in glomerular basement membrane and the walls of blood vessels. In the rabbit model, IgE antibody may have an important role in this respect: interaction of antigen with cell-bound IgE is followed by the release of platelet-aggregating factor which triggers the release of histamine and other mediators from platelets. The vasoactive effects of these substances are believed to encourage the subsequent localization of IgG-containing immune complexes. Early treatment with

antagonists of vasoactive amines is claimed to inhibit the development of arteritis and glomerulonephritis in the acute serum sickness model, while glomerulonephritis in the chronic model is prevented largely, and established nephritis improved, by such measures.

One recent study has shown that the immunosuppressive drug cyclosporin A can inhibit the glomerular proliferation and proteinuria seen in acute serum sickness. Since cyclosporin A is thought to act preferentially on proliferating T cells, the finding implies that T cells may play a role in mediating glomerular damage.

Clinical detection of immune complexes

The contribution of immune complex deposition to the clinical features of a disease is usually assessed in two ways: one approach is the analysis of tissue specimens for direct evidence of complex deposition and the other is the identification of complexes in serum or body fluids.

Biopsy evidence

Direct immunofluorescence of tissue biopsies is of considerable value: in practice, kidney and skin are the most commonly biopsied sites and interpretation of the changes seen in these organs is more helpful than for biopsies of other tissues. Biopsies should be placed in saline and taken directly to the laboratory where they are snap-frozen and sectioned in a cryostat. Components of immune complexes can be identified by incubating the sections with fluorescein-labelled antisera specific for human immunoglobulins, complement or even the suspected antigen.

Immunoglobulin or complement deposition in a pattern similar to that seen in experimentally induced immune complex disease provides indirect evidence that immune complexes are responsible for the clinical symptoms in the patient under investigation. Definitive proof of this assumption depends on demonstrating the presence of antigen in the complexes and eluting an antibody from affected tissue which reacts specifically with this antigen. In practice, such proof is usually lacking.

Skin biopsies

Immune complexes in the blood vessels and at the dermoepidermal junction (DEJ) of the skin have been found in a wide variety of localized and systemic diseases (*Table 5.3*). Skin biopsy is of value in distinguishing between SLE and discoid lupus erythematosus (DLE).

Table 5.3 Conditions associated with immune complex deposition in skin[a]

Disease	Deposit
SLE	} IgG, C3 (usually), IgA,
DLE	} IgM, C4, factor B (often)
Dermatitis herpetiformis	IgA, C3
Lepromatous leprosy	IgG, IgM, C3
Cutaneous vasculitis	IgG, IgM, C3

[a]Biospy of clinically *uninvolved* skin is of diagnostic value in patients with suspected dermatitis herpetiformis or SLE

Figure 5.9 *Direct immunofluorescent examination of a biopsy of clinically unaffected skin in SLE. Granular deposition of IgG is seen at the dermoepidermal junction*

Figure 5.10 *Granular deposition of IgA in the dermal papillae of clinically normal skin in dermatitis herpetiformis*

Coarse, granular, irregular deposits of immunoglobulin (particularly IgG) and complement are seen along the DEJ of most biopsied lesions in both SLE and DLE. In contrast, a similar pattern is found in clinically unaffected skin from most patients with active SLE (*Figure 5.9*) but not those with DLE and forms the basis of the so-called 'lupus band test'.

In dermatitis herpetiformis (DH), clinically normal skin shows characteristic granular deposits of IgA and C3 in the dermal papillae (*Figure 5.10*) but, surprisingly, affected skin fails to show this pattern. The known relationship between DH and coeliac disease suggests that circulating complexes of dietary gluten and antigluten antibody may be involved. Dapsone (Maloprim), which is of benefit in DH, blocks the effects of experimentally induced immune complex disease.

Renal biopsies

In man, immune complex deposition is assumed to be responsible for the overwhelming majority of cases of glomerulonephritis. Although the list of suggested exogenous and endogenous antigens is extensive (*see Table 5.1*), these offending antigens have rarely been identified within the complex itself.

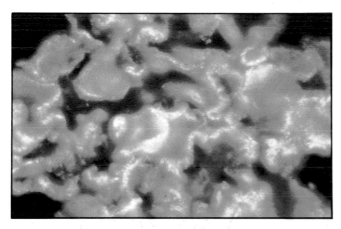

Figure 5.11 *The glomerulus of a patient with SLE. Granular deposits of IgG are present along the glomerular capillary wall. A similar staining pattern was seen in this biopsy with fluorescein-labelled antisera to IgM, C3 and C4*

Immune complex nephritis is typified by granular deposition of IgG and C3 in the glomerulus (*Figure 5.11*). In SLE, labelled antisera to IgM, IgA, C1q, C4 and properdin may also show a similar staining pattern, suggesting activation of both the classical and alternative complement pathways: this generalized pattern of staining is character-

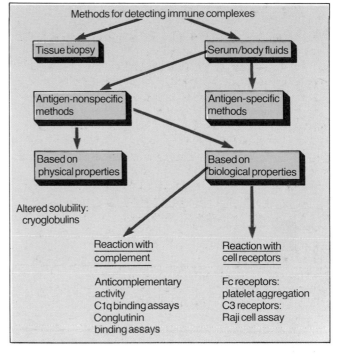

Figure 5.12 *Classification of selected methods for detecting immune complexes*

istic of renal lupus and rarely found in other conditions. These deposits have been eluted from diseased kidneys and shown to consist of DNA, other nuclear antigens and antibodies to these proteins. During remission, or in the absence of overt renal involvement, staining is usually slight and confined to the mesangium; in active renal lupus, however, there are heavy deposits throughout the glomerulus, including the epithelial basement membrane.

Acute poststreptococcal glomerulonephritis shows many similarities to 'one-shot' serum sickness. There is granular deposition of IgG, C3 and occasionally IgM along the glomerular basement membrane in association with electron-dense subepithelial deposits. Streptococcal cell wall material is detectable in glomeruli by immunofluorescence but only at the very beginning of the inflammatory process.

Table 5.4 Limitations of selected tests for immune complexes

Principle	Assay	Component detected	Interfering substances	Sensitivity
Physical properties	Cryoprecipitation	?	Aggregated IgG	+
Reactivity with complement	Anticomplementary activity	IgG, IgM	Aggregated IgG DNA Endotoxin C-reactive protein	+++
	C1q binding assays	IgG, IgM	Aggregated IgG ? DNA ? Endotoxin	++
	Conglutinin binding assays	IgG, IgM	Aggregated IgG	+++
Binding to cell receptors for activated C3	Raji cell radioimmunoassay	C3b	Aggregated IgG Antilymphocyte antibodies Antinuclear antibodies	+++
Binding to Fc receptors	Platelet aggregation	IgG	Aggregated IgG Antiplatelet antibodies Some viruses	+++

Tests for circulating immune complexes

Available assays (*Figure 5.12*) either identify complexes in a nonspecific fashion or selectively pick up complexes containing a particular antigen. Such antigen-specific methods have allowed the demonstration of circulating complexes containing DNA, insulin, hepatitis B and dietary antigens in the sera of some individuals.

In recent years there has been a proliferation of methods reported to detect circulating immune complexes: all have their advocates. The methods are based on the distinct properties of complexed immunoglobulin molecules compared with free immunoglobulin: essentially these are *physical* properties resulting from the formation of a complex of large molecular weight and *biological* properties such as complement fixation or binding to cell-membrane receptors. Most immunology laboratories offer one or more of the methods shown (*Table 5.4*) but the list is not intended to be exhaustive.

Limitations of immune complex assays

The underlying principle of a test imposes limitations on its capacity to detect immune complexes (*Table 5.4*). The basis of cryoprecipitation is not fully understood; this method detects only some complexes. Complement-receptor-dependent tests will not detect complexes that fail to activate and bind complement because of the size of the complex or its antibody component, while C1q binding assays will miss complexes of IgA or IgE. Fc receptor tests (for example, platelet aggregation) cannot detect complexes containing immunoglobulins other than IgG.

It should also be appreciated that all methods are subject to some interference from substances other than immune complexes and that, unfortunately, no method is able to distinguish nonspecifically aggregated immunoglobulins from true immune complexes. Inadequate storage of sera, or repeated freezing and thawing of samples, causes immunoglobulins to aggregate and thus may generate

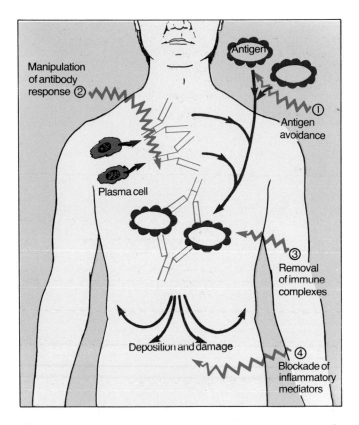

Figure 5.13 *Approaches to the treatment of immune complex disorders: these include elimination of the antigen (1); manipulation of the quality of antibody produced (2); removal of circulating immune complexes (3) and blockade of inflammatory mediators (4)*

false-positive results. There is also a considerable difference in the pattern of reactivity of sera from patients with different diseases in these various tests: the basis for this difference is not understood. It is clear, however, that a number of tests, particularly the C1q binding assays, conglutinin-binding assay, Raji cell assay and platelet aggregation test, do distinguish pathological from normal sera and that positive results in these assays strongly suggest the presence of immune complexes.

Approach to the treatment of immune complex diseases

Most forms of treatment for immune complex diseases are aimed at producing relief of symptoms or at counteracting the effects of tissue injury rather than reversing the underlying process of complex deposition.

Patients with immune complex diseases seem poor at handling complexes: this may be because of the nature of the antigen component or the quality of the antibody produced, or because of a dysfunction of their MPS and complement system. A logical and direct approach to the treatment of immune complex diseases can therefore be divided into four main categories (*Figure 5.13*): antigen elimination, removal of circulating formed complexes, manipulation of the antibody response, and modulation of inflammatory mediators.

Antigen elimination

Although the antigen is unknown in most cases of immune complex disease, occasionally it is feasible to remove the offending antigen. In the case of an identifiable micro-organism, as in immune complex disease associated with malaria, schistosomiasis or infected ventriculoatrial shunts, direct benefit can be obtained by treatment of the primary infection. Similarly, immune complex damage resulting from drug hypersensitivity can be minimized by recognition and avoidance of the drug. In DH, dietary gluten withdrawal undoubtedly improves the associated jejunal villous atrophy but there is disagreement as to whether or not the skin lesions are improved by this measure alone.

An alternative but experimental approach is directed at the removal of circulating antigen using extracorporeal immunoabsorbents. For example, anti-DNA antibodies linked to an immunoabsorbent column will bind free DNA, so removing the circulating antigen and altering the antigen–antibody ratio. If DNA is linked to the immuno-absorbent, then anti-DNA antibodies may be removed from the plasma of patients with SLE.

Removal of immune complexes

A second, major approach is the use of plasma exchange to remove circulating, soluble immune complexes. There are many potential benefits from this approach (*Table 5.5*). The additional removal of free antigen would alter both the rate of formation of immune complexes and the antigen–antibody ratio which determines the size and lattice structure of the complexes.

Table 5.5 Potential benefits of plasma exchange

Removal of immune-complex load

Removal of free antigen

Removal of low-affinity antibody

Alteration of antigen–antibody ratio

Reversal of blockade of MPS

Removal of nonspecific inflammatory mediators

In some cases, persistence of immune complexes implies a functional impairment of the MPS arising either because the amount of soluble complexes generated exceeds the capacity of the MPS to clear them, or because there is a primary defect of MPS function. Plasma exchange under these circumstances can produce partial reversal of MPS blockade.

In-vitro studies suggest that complement can solubilize preformed immune complexes. This property may be impaired in some diseases (such as SLE) associated with marked consumption of complement, but restored following plasma exchange.

Some immune disorders have been treated successfully by plasma exchange (*Table 5.6*). The place of plasma exchange compared with conventional treatment and its role and timing in individual cases remain to be established firmly. Nevertheless, plasma exchange appears to be a relatively safe procedure with few side-effects. Reported hazards include allergic reactions to replacement fluid and plasma, transmission of hepatitis, transient thrombocytopenia, disordered fluid balance, citrate toxicity and

Table 5.6 Immune complex mediated diseases successfully treated by plasma exchange

SLE

Rapidly progressive glomerulonephritis
  Wegener's granulomatosis
  Polyarteritis nodosa

Mixed essential cryoglobulinaemia

Cutaneous vasculitis

coagulation disorders following exchange, and local infection at the sites of arteriovenous access.

Manipulation of the immune response

Evidence from experimental models has led to the broad concept that immune complexes persist in poor (low-affinity) antibody formers but not in those who either produce high-affinity antibody or who fail to produce any antibody.

Immunosuppressive agents used in diseases of this type, such as corticosteroids or cytotoxic drugs, exert some of their beneficial effects by impairing humoral antibody production, so indirectly limiting the formation of circulating complexes. Plasma exchange may also be immunosuppressive in transforming a poor antibody former into one who produces virtually no antibody at all, with beneficial effect.

A more novel alternative would be to stimulate the immune system to generate high-affinity antibody capable of allowing the efficient clearance of immune complexes.

Modulation of inflammatory mediators

Many factors, including platelet-derived substances and various vasoactive amines, may facilitate immune complex deposition and subsequent inflammation. These effects could be reduced by modifying the processes of blood coagulation, platelet adhesiveness, prostaglandin synthesis or functional complement activity by the judicious use of immunosuppressive drugs. In experimental chronic immune complex glomerulonephritis, prior platelet depletion or administration of potent inhibitors of platelet vasoactive amines can markedly reduce vascular inflammation and complex deposition. The presence of fibrin or fibrinogen-related material in affected tissues has suggested that the clotting system may be a primary mediator of damage in immune complex nephritis; there is, however, no direct evidence in support of this hypothesis.

Clinical implications of the detection of immune complexes

The major pathological features of some conditions seem convincingly related to the formation and tissue deposition of complexes, complexes of DNA/anti-DNA antibody in SLE being the classical example. The availability of sensitive immune complex assays has demonstrated that circulating complexes are also present in low levels in people without apparent disease; therefore, not all immune complexes are damaging. The finding of immune complexes in pathological samples must always be interpreted with this observation in mind. For immune complexes to be considered of fundamental importance in the pathogenesis of a disease, certain criteria should be fulfilled (*Table 5.7*). In conditions meeting these criteria, the quantitation of circulating complexes may be of practical value in follow-up.

In other disorders, the formation of immune complexes may be a secondary event occurring during the course of the disease, but may still account for some of the pathological manifestations, such as in poststreptococcal glomerulonephritis.

Table 5.7 Criteria necessary to substantiate an immune complex aetiology

Are immune complexes present at sites of tissue damage?

Are immune complexes detectable in the circulation?

What is the nature of the immune complex? (Can the antigen component be identified?)

Does removal of immune complexes produce clinical improvement?

A third group includes those conditions in which immune complexes are found without obvious direct pathological consequences. Even so, such complexes still might exert a subtle effect on cell function that cannot be detected by existing techniques.

Further reading

ALLEN, B. R. and REEVES, W. G. (1983) Skin diseases. In *Immunology in Medicine*, 2nd edn (E. J. Holborow and W. G. Reeves, eds). Academic Press, London

MANNICK, M. (1982) Pathophysiology of circulating immune complexes. *Arthritis and Rheumatism*, **25**, 783–787

NEILD, G. H., IVORY, K., HIRAMATSU, M. and WILLIAMS, D. G. (1983) Cyclosporin A inhibits acute serum sickness in rabbits. *Clinical and Experimental Immunology*, **52**, 586–594

PINCHING, A. J. (1980) Plasma exchange in immunologically mediated disease. In *Recent Advances in Clinical Immunology*, vol. 2 (R. A. Thompson, ed). Churchill Livingstone, Edinburgh

SUTTON, D. H. C., CARDELLA, C. J., ULDALL, P. R., et al. (1981) Complications of intensive plasma exchange. *Plasma Therapy*, **2**, 19–24

ZUBLER, R. H. and LAMBERT, P. H. (1977) Immune complexes in clinical investigation. In *Recent Advances in Clinical Immunology*, vol. 1 (R. A. Thompson, ed.) Churchill Livingstone, Edinburgh

6 Antibody deficiency

Resistance to an infection depends upon many factors, including not only the balance between natural immunity and the virulence of the infecting organism but also the effectiveness of nonspecific defences such as the skin and mucosal surfaces, the expulsive action of bronchial cilia, the action of bactericidal substances such as lysozyme and the maintenance of local pH conditions.

Breakdown of local mechanical barriers, for example by severe burns, is invariably accompanied by impaired resistance to infection in spite of intact immune responses. If microorganisms successfully evade these barriers, their elimination then requires cooperation between elements of the immune system. Unfortunately, in some individuals, defective immunity predisposes them to persistent, recurrent or unusual infections.

Cellular basis of defective immunity

Specific immunity is conventionally classified into humoral immunity and cell-mediated immunity. By definition, non-specific immune mechanisms lack immunological memory of the antigen, yet defects of these pathways, which include the phagocyte and complement systems, are also accompanied by severe infections.

Specific immune mechanisms

Studies of the immune system in the chicken and the mouse have shown the existence of at least two distinct subpopulations of lymphocytes, termed T and B lympho-

cytes. These cells follow analogous maturation pathways (*Figure 6.1*). They are derived from a common bone-marrow stem cell which gives rise to cells precommitted to entering a particular tissue environment. This tissue induces pre-B or pre-T cells to differentiate into B or T cells equipped with cell-surface receptors for specific recognition of antigen and for cooperation with other cells. Then, when triggered by the appropriate stimulus, T and B lymphocytes undergo terminal differentiation to effector cells and a pool of memory cells which retain the capacity to generate further

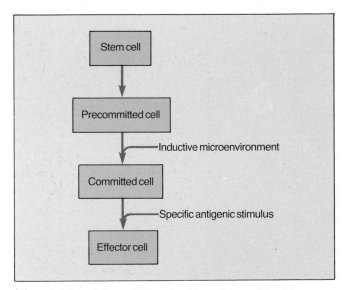

Figure 6.1 *Essential steps in the maturation pathways of T and B lymphocytes*

progeny on subsequent stimulation by the original antigen. Whereas the life of an effector cell is measured in days, memory cells may survive for years.

T lymphocytes

Maturation of T cells occurs within the microenvironment of the thymus, which remains functional throughout life in spite of a considerable reduction in size after puberty. T lymphocytes leaving the thymus enter predetermined T cell areas of peripheral lymphoid tissue. Exposure of mature T lymphocytes to antigen generates several types of effector cells (*Figure 6.2*).

Helper T cells (T_H)

These cooperate with B lymphocytes in the induction of antibody responses. Macrophages are also required but are not antigen-specific; their function can be performed by appropriate cells from a nonimmunized host. In contrast, antigen-specific T_H and B cells must both be present to produce an antibody response; this explains why patients with severely impaired cell-mediated immunity (and hence poor T_H activity) may also have poor antibody responses.

Suppressor T cells (T_S)

These limit the extent to which the host responds to antigenic stimulation and have an important regulatory effect on both antibody and cell-mediated immune responses. Helper and suppressor subpopulations of T cells can be distinguished by monoclonal antibodies which recognize different cell surface characteristics and also by *in-vitro* functional assays.

Cytotoxic T cells (T_C)

These are specifically sensitized to kill foreign cells bearing the appropriate antigens, provided that the killer and target cells share the same histocompatibility antigens. Cytotoxic T cells are particularly important in host defence against viral infections.

B lymphocytes

In birds, B lymphocyte induction occurs in the bursa of Fabricius, a lymphoid pouch that connects with the hind gut. It was this finding that gave rise to the designation of 'B' for 'bursal' cells. In mammals, the equivalent microen-

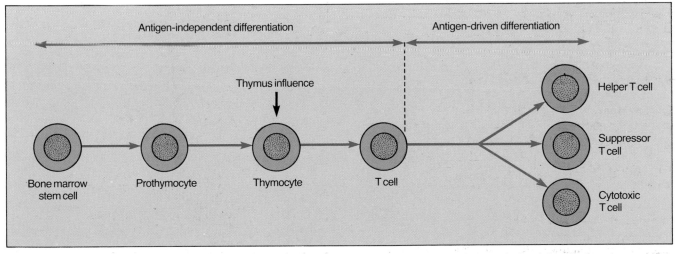

Figure 6.2 *Maturation of T lymphocytes. Antigen-independent maturation of T cells in the thymus generates a population of short-lived, antigen-specific T cells. Those T cells that meet specific antigen differentiate into effector T cells*

vironment is believed to reside in the liver and perhaps the spleen in fetal life, and in the bone marrow in adult life.

During maturation, cells of the B lineage acquire stage-specific cell-surface receptors which can be used clinically as markers, for example in the typing of leukaemic cells. B cells leaving the bone marrow 'home' to predetermined B cell areas of peripheral lymphoid tissue. These cells are probably short-lived: like virgin T cells, they are believed to require stimulation by specific antigen to trigger further differentiation to mature long-lived, recirculating B cells. These respond to further antigenic stimulation by terminal differentiation into memory B cells and antibody-secreting plasma cells (*Figure 6.3*).

Nonspecific immune mechanisms

Macrophages are essential for the induction of most antibody and cell-mediated immune responses (*Figure 6.4*). Phagocytic cells take up antigens in a nonspecific manner: while most of the ingested material is degraded, the macrophage cell surface retains or receives a small amount of highly immunogenic material for presentation to antigen-specific T and B lymphocytes. In addition, macrophages enable effective collaboration between lymphocyte subpopulations.

Normal humoral immunity depends not only upon the differentiation of B cells into antibody-producing plasma cells but also upon effector mechanisms which then eliminate bound antigen (*Figure 6.5*). Thus complement-dependent lysis of bacteria requires a functioning complement system as well as synthesis of complement-fixing IgM or IgG antibodies. Foreign particles coated (opsonized) with IgG antibodies are readily bound and ingested by phagocytic cells. Thus specific immunity needs nonspecific effector mechanisms to be fully operative: this interdependence partly explains the basic similarities between the types of infections experienced by patients with defects of either antibody synthesis or phagocyte function.

Basic classification of immunodeficiency

Defective immunity can be classified into primary or secondary disorders involving either specific or nonspecific immune mechanisms (*Figure 6.6*). However, in

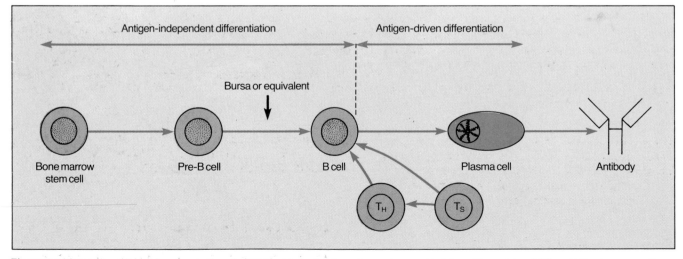

Figure 6.3 *Maturation of B lymphocytes. Antigen-independent induction in a microenvironment is followed by peripheral differentiation to memory B cells and antibody-secreting plasma cells. The development of mature plasma cells after antigen-triggering of B cells takes about five days and eight cell generations.*

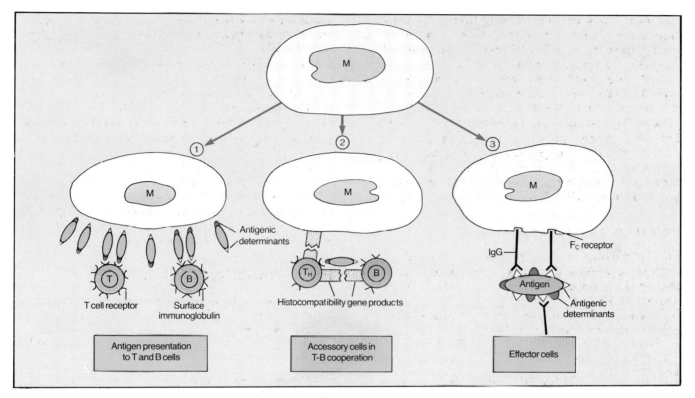

Figure 6.4 *The functions of phagocytic cells. (1) Macrophages concentrate antigen for presentation to antigen-specific receptors on T and B lymphocytes. These receptors recognize different determinants on the same molecule. (2) Macrophages are required as accessory cells during the efficient cooperation between T and B lymphocytes. Additional cell surface receptors, the products of genes sited in the MHC, may also be involved in regulation of the immune response to a given antigen. (3) Phagocytic cells rapidly ingest and degrade antigens which have been coated with IgG antibody or the activated third component of complement, C3b*

some studies, up to half of all patients with clinical suspicion of immunodeficiency are 'normal' by existing laboratory techniques, while most of the remainder show subtle or transient abnormalities. In only a few can the defect be classified into defined syndromes.

Primary antibody deficiency

Defects in antibody synthesis are qualitative or quantitative: quantitative defects may involve all immunoglobulin classes (panhypogammaglobulinaemia) or only one class (or subclass) of immunoglobulin (selective deficiency). A World Health Organization classification (*Table 6.1*) is widely used.

Diagnosis and assessment of defect in antibody synthesis

The patient's history and examination is of prime importance because laboratory tests never entirely exclude minor degrees of immunodeficiency. The history helps to

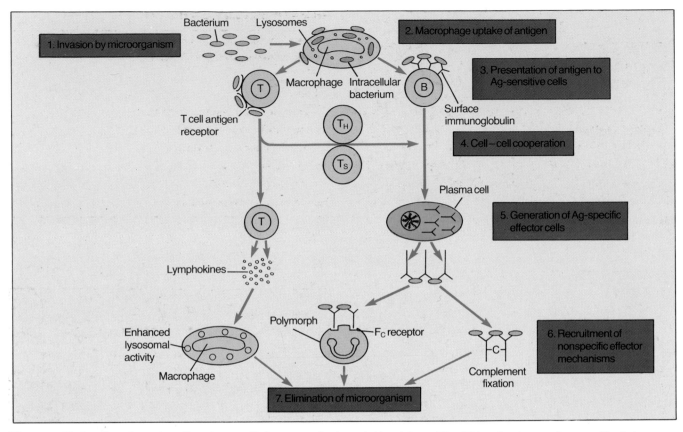

Figure 6.5 *The interdependence of specific and nonspecific immune mechanisms. Antigen-triggered T and B lymphocytes recruit nonspecific effector mechanisms to eliminate the antigen. These mechanisms include complement-dependent lysis and enhanced phagocytosis of antigen by polymorphs and macrophages*

distinguish relatively rare primary immunodeficiencies from more common secondary causes of recurrent infections: for example, inhaled foreign bodies or cystic fibrosis are much more likely causes of recurrent chest infections in childhood than are immunodeficiency states.

Clues from the history

Antibody deficiency should be suspected in any patient with persistent, recurrent, severe or unusual infections, bearing in mind that presentation can occur at any age.

Presenting symptoms

Recurrent infections of the upper and lower respiratory tracts occur in almost all patients (*Figure 6.7*). Many patients additionally suffer from skin sepsis (boils and cellulitis) or meningitis.

Age of onset

Infants with congenital hypogammaglobulinaemia are partly protected by maternally transferred IgG for the first 3–4 months of life. In this group, recurrent infections tend

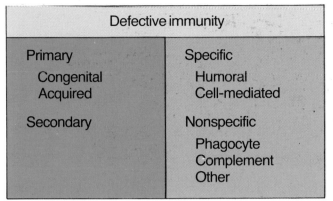

Figure 6.6 *Basic classification of defects in immune function*

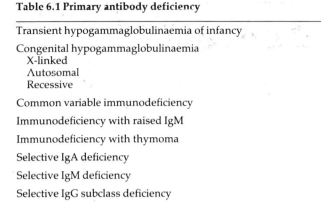

Table 6.1 Primary antibody deficiency

Transient hypogammaglobulinaemia of infancy

Congenital hypogammaglobulinaemia
    X-linked
    Autosomal
    Recessive

Common variable immunodeficiency

Immunodeficiency with raised IgM

Immunodeficiency with thymoma

Selective IgA deficiency

Selective IgM deficiency

Selective IgG subclass deficiency

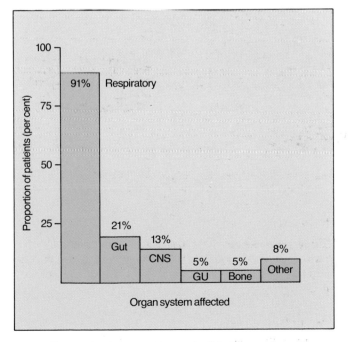
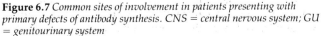

Figure 6.7 *Common sites of involvement in patients presenting with primary defects of antibody synthesis. CNS = central nervous system; GU = genitourinary system*

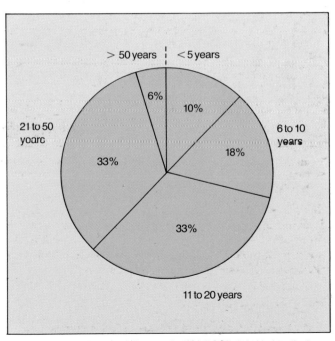

Figure 6.8 *Age at diagnosis of patients with primary defects of antibody synthesis*

to occur between the ages of 6 months and 2 years. However, most patients with antibody deficiency present in the second decade or later (*Figure 6.8*).

Family history

A few types of primary antibody deficiency are inherited as X-linked recessive or autosomal recessive traits and in these patients a history of affected relatives is of diagnostic value. However, the average family size is now so small that a negative family history does not exclude an inherited condition.

Nature of pathogens

Pyogenic organisms such as staphylococci, streptococci, *Haemophilus influenzae* and pneumococci are the commonest pathogens in antibody deficiency syndromes. In general, these patients are not unduly susceptible to viral or fungal infections.

Clues from the examination

There are rarely any diagnostic physical signs of antibody deficiency, although examination often reveals evidence of previous severe infections and their consequences, such as bronchiectasis. A common feature of children with antibody deficiency is a failure to thrive, and serial plotting of height and weight is a useful guide to the effectiveness of therapy (*Figure 6.9*).

Laboratory tests

Serum immunoglobulin levels

Measurement of serum immunoglobulin levels will reveal any gross quantitative abnormality of immunoglobulin classes. A complete absence of immunoglobulin (agammaglobulinaemia) is unusual, and even severely affected patients have detectable levels of IgG and IgM (that is, hypogammaglobulinaemia). Interpretation of serum immunoglobulin levels must always be related to the age of the patient.

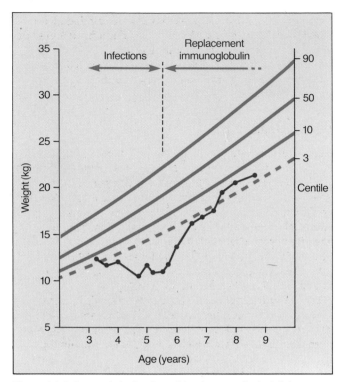

Figure 6.9 *Failure to thrive in a boy with primary antibody deficiency. Immunoglobulin replacement therapy was accompanied by gradual weight gain*

Secretory immunoglobulin levels

IgA is the main immunoglobulin in secretions, where it exists as two molecules bound to a protein called secretory piece which protects secretory IgA from proteolytic digestion. Quantitation of secretory IgA and free secretory piece in samples of saliva will detect most patients with major defects of this local immune system although there are many technical problems associated with accurate measurement of secretory immunoglobulins.

Functional antibody activity

The ability of a patient to make antibody is a better guide to his susceptibility to infection than total serum immunoglobulin levels. Some individuals have been described who failed to make specific antibody after immunization in spite of normal serum immunoglobulin levels.

Tests for functional antibody include the detection of naturally occurring antibody activity and the response to test immunization.

Natural antibodies

Useful natural antibodies in this context are serum isohaemagglutinins to blood group substances A and B and antibodies produced against gut commensals such as *Escherichia coli*. Isohaemagglutinins are usually of IgM class and the titre slowly increases over the first 2 years of life. Although there is a wide variation in the final titre, the absence of serum isoagglutinins in a patient of the appropriate blood group is likely to be significant. Interpretation may be less clear-cut in infants in whom isoagglutinin activity is not fully developed.

Using erythrocytes coated with pooled antigen from several *E. coli* serotypes, haemagglutinating antibodies can be detected in high titre (>1/32) in the sera of virtually all normal subjects: the antibodies are again predominantly of IgM class.

In individuals who have been naturally exposed to common infections, measurement of complement-fixing antibodies to a panel of viral antigens or measurement of antistreptolysin 0 titres provides an assessment of the capacity to synthesize antibodies. The screening laboratory must, of course, be informed of the purpose of the request so that the serum can be tested at dilutions different to those appropriate for diagnosis of an acute viral infection.

Test immunization

Patients with suspected or proven defects in antibody production should not be immunized with 'live' vaccines: there are several examples of disseminated infection following immunization. The theoretical advantages of test immunization must be weighed against the ethical difficulties of selecting a safe antigen. One exception is the bacteriophage φX174: this DNA virus is generally accepted as safe because it replicates only in one serotype of *E. coli*

and does not infect mammalian cells. Test immunization with φX174 produces classical primary (IgM) and secondary (IgG) antibody responses in normal individuals. Tetanus toxoid and polyvalent pneumococcal vaccine (Pneumovax) also produce good IgG antibody responses and distinguish normal subjects from those with impaired antibody production.

Circulating B lymphocyte numbers

Circulating B lymphocytes are usually defined by the presence of surface membrane immunoglobulin (SmIg) (*Figure 6.10*). In normal blood, SmIg-positive cells constitute 5–15% of the total lymphocyte population. Although counting numbers of B lymphocytes in various diseases is generally of doubtful clinical value, the absence of B cells in an immunodeficient patient distinguishes congenital X-linked hypogammaglobulinaemia from other causes of antibody deficiency in which normal or low numbers of circulating B cells are found.

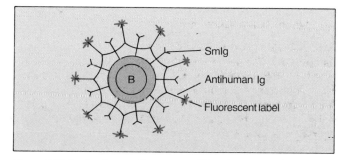

Figure 6.10 *Surface immunofluorescence. B lymphocytes are characterized by surface immunoglobulin molecules inserted in the cell membrane which function as the antigen receptors. Surface membrane immunoglobulin (SmIg) can be detected by adding a fluorescein-labelled antibody to human immunoglobulin*

Causes of primary antibody deficiency (*Table 6.1*)

Transient hypogammaglobulinaemia of infancy

Maternal IgG is normally transferred across the placenta to the fetus from the fourth month of gestational life onwards but maximum transfer occurs during the last 4 weeks. The newborn infant thus has a serum IgG level similar to that of the mother. Other immunoglobulin classes are not transferred and elevated levels of IgM or IgA in cord blood suggest specific antibody synthesis in response to intrauterine infection.

At birth, therefore, serum IgG is wholly maternal in origin (*Figure 6.11*): catabolism of this transferred IgG is only partly compensated by endogenous IgG production. The period between 3 and 6 months of age represents a phase of 'physiological hypogammaglobulinaemia' although the infant is not unduly susceptible to infection because functioning antibody is present in spite of the lower total IgG level. The trough in IgG is more severe when the amount of IgG acquired from the mother is reduced, as in prematurity.

Transient hypogammaglobulinaemia thus defines a condition in which the infant is slower than usual to synthesize IgG: as serum levels of maternally transferred IgG fall further, the infant becomes susceptible to recurrent pyogenic infections. After several months or more (up to 1–2 years), spontaneous IgG production begins and serum IgG levels slowly rise.

Management

It is important to distinguish this condition from pathological causes of hypogammaglobulinaemia because the treatment differs. In most cases, the infant remains well, apart from mild upper respiratory tract infections, and no specific treatment is needed: however, serum immunoglobulin levels should be remeasured at intervals of about 3

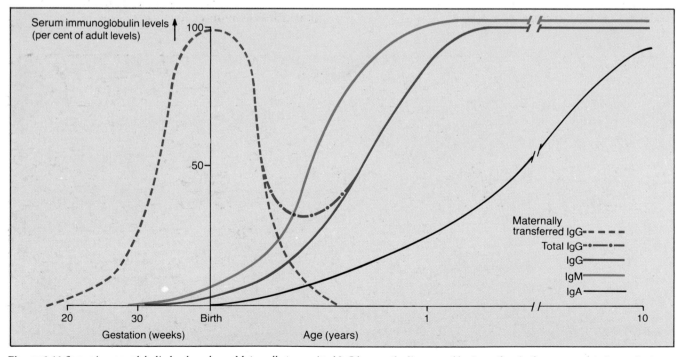

Figure 6.11 *Serum immunoglobulin levels and age. Maternally transmitted IgG has mostly disappeared by 6 months. As the neonate actively synthesizes IgG the level slowly rises, but a physiological trough of serum IgG is characteristically seen at 3–6 months*

months. If infections are severe, then replacement immunoglobulins will prevent further morbidity. The dose of immunoglobulins is the same as that for other causes of antibody deficiency (see below). Treatment may be needed for 1–2 years but can be discontinued when there is clinical improvement with rising immunoglobulin levels and detectable specific antibody activity.

Infantile sex-linked hypogammaglobulinaemia (Bruton's disease)

Boys with this condition usually present with recurrent pyogenic infections at the age of 6 months to 2 years. The sites of infection, and the organisms involved are similar to other types of antibody deficiency (*Figure 6.7*). Such children usually handle viral infections, for example measles and varicella, without difficulty. There are no distinctive physical findings.

Diagnosis

The diagnosis rests on the very low serum levels of all classes of immunoglobulins together with a family history of affected male relatives. Sometimes, however, a convincing genetic pattern is lacking.

Immunology

In almost all patients, circulating B lymphocytes are absent but T cells are normal or even increased. No plasma cells are found in the bone marrow, lymph nodes or gastrointestinal tract. These findings argue in favour of a defect of the microenvironment needed for B lymphocyte induction (*Figure 6.12*), although the exact mechanism is unknown. The absence of circulating B cells distinguishes this condition from transient hypogammaglobulinaemia of infancy and other causes of antibody deficiency. Studies of cell-mediated immunity are usually normal.

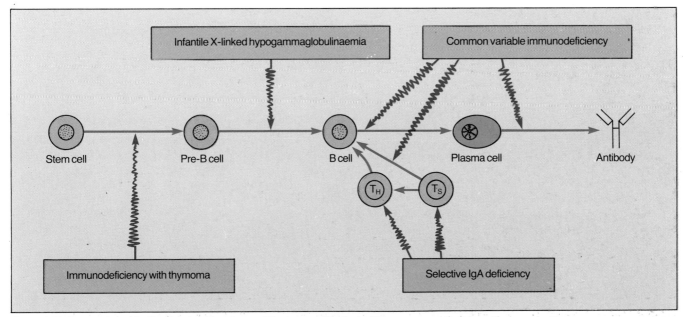

Figure 6.12 *An overview of the B cell maturation steps and the presumed levels at which commoner defects in antibody production occur*

Hypogammaglobulinaemia with IgM

Some children with very low serum levels of IgG and IgA have normal or raised levels of IgM: most are boys with affected male relatives, suggesting an X-linked recessive mode of inheritance but there is also a form which affects both sexes.

Low or normal numbers of B cells with surface IgM are present, suggesting that the defect is one of maturation of antigen-responsive B lymphocytes. Unfortunately, the IgM present seems to have little significant antibody activity.

Treatment is similar to that of other forms of antibody deficiency but paradoxically the high serum IgM levels may fall during the course of regular immunoglobulin replacement therapy.

Common variable immunodeficiency

This category embraces a heterogeneous group of disorders presenting in childhood or adult life. Males and females are affected in approximately equal proportions, with a prevalence in Britain of about 10 per million of the population. Some patients have affected relatives.

Clinical features

The features depend on the severity of the antibody deficiency. Severely affected individuals experience the same range of infections as other patients with antibody deficiency (*Figure 6.7*). Symptoms can occur at any age although most patients become symptomatic in the second to fourth decades (*Figure 6.8*).

Patients may suffer a wide range of complications (*see below*) but many survive to middle age or beyond. Women with this disorder have given birth to normal offspring, although the infants were naturally hypogammaglobulinaemic for the first 6 months of life.

Immunology

Most patients have very low serum levels of IgG, IgA and IgM, with normal or only slightly decreased numbers of circulating B and T lymphocytes. About 60–70% of patients have intact cell-mediated immunity but the remainder demonstrate variable abnormalities, including impaired delayed hypersensitivity skin reactions to common antigens and depressed lymphocyte transformation responses to mitogens. Lymph nodes usually lack germinal centres, and immunoglobulin-containing lymphoid cells and plasma cells are rarely present other than in the lamina propria of the gut.

Pathogenesis

Several patterns of variable immunodeficiency are apparent. In some individuals there is a defect of differentiation into antibody-secreting plasma cells (*Figure 6.12*). This category includes patients whose cells can be stimulated to produce, but not secrete, immunoglobulin *in vitro* and who may have a defect in intracellular glycosylation of the immunoglobulin molecule.

In other patients there is defective immunoregulation: thus, their B cells will differentiate into immunoglobulin-secreting cells when cultured in the presence of normal T cells but not their own T cells. Conversely, T cells from this group of patients can suppress the differentiation and immunoglobulin synthesis of normal lymphocytes, suggesting that the primary defect involves T cell suppression of essentially normal B lymphocytes (*Figure 6.12*). This evidence has been challenged: it has been shown in other experiments that *in-vitro* immunoglobulin production by B cells is abnormal in most of these patients even when incubated with normal T cells in optimal ratios. Failure of immunoglobulin synthesis may be caused by loss of the normal mature circulating B cell or by its replacement by early B cells of the type found in the bone marrow. It is also possible that the suppressor cells which depress immunoglobulin production *in vitro* also depress B cell development in the bone marrow. In contrast, helper T cell function appears to be normal in patients with this condition.

Immunodeficiency with thymoma

This condition involves a defect of B cell development characterized by hypogammaglobulinaemia associated with thymoma: in many cases, abnormal T cell function is also found.

Clinical features

Most patients present between 40 and 70 years of age with recurrent respiratory tract infections, but some also suffer from chronic mucocutaneous candidiasis or cytomegalovirus infection. A proportion have associated haematological disorders: about one third of patients have a pure red cell aplasia characteristic of thymoma and some lack circulating and bone-marrow eosinophils.

The thymoma tends to be of the spindle cell variety and is usually benign or only locally invasive. The cause-and-effect relationship of hypogammaglobulinaemia with the thymoma is not clear as removal of the thymoma does not produce any improvement in the immunodeficiency.

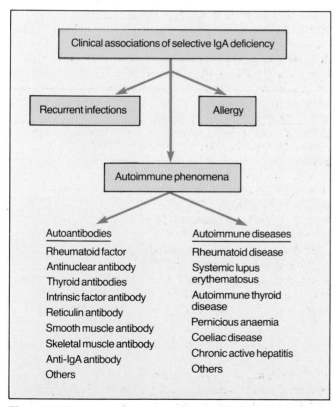

Figure 6.13 *Disorders commonly reported in association with selective IgA deficiency*

Immunology

Serum immunoglobulin levels are rarely as low as in other forms of panhypogammaglobulinaemia and there is a variable antibody response to specific immunization. *In-vitro* tests of cell-mediated immunity are abnormal in about half of cases.

Pathogenesis

In contrast to patients with common variable immunodeficiency, patients with hypogammaglobulinaemia and thymoma lack marrow pre-B cells and have absent or very low numbers of circulating B lymphocytes, suggesting that the fundamental defect, although undefined, involves impaired transformation of marrow stem cells into cells of the B line (*Figure 6.12*).

Selective IgA deficiency

This condition is characterized by undetectable serum IgA levels with normal levels of IgG and IgM. It is the commonest primary defect of specific immunity, with an incidence of approximately 1 in 700 in the UK.

Clinical features

Most IgA-deficient people identified by screening of blood donors are healthy: nevertheless, selective IgA deficiency does appear to predispose the individual to a variety of disorders (*Figure 6.13*).

Recurrent infections

These usually involve either the upper respiratory tract (causing otitis media, sinusitis and bronchitis) or the gut (in the form of recurrent diarrhoea caused mainly by small intestinal bacterial overgrowth). Yet most selective IgA deficient individuals are asymptomatic because IgM, which is produced in normal amounts, can bind to secretory piece and substitute for secretory IgA at mucosal surfaces.

Allergy and IgA deficiency

Selective IgA deficiency is said to be commoner in atopic patients than in the normal population. While the reasons for this association are not entirely clear, circulating antibodies to dietary antigens, especially cow's milk, have been found in about half of patients. This finding suggests that the lack of IgA in mucosal secretions leads to increased intestinal permeability and excessive absorption of many food proteins, resulting in formation of antigen-antibody complexes or stimulation of IgE synthesis.

About one-third of patients with selective IgA deficiency make antibodies to IgA in the absence of any previous transfusion history. Some of these subsequently develop anaphylactic reactions after transfusion of plasma or blood.

Autoimmunity and IgA deficiency

Patients with selective IgA deficiency have an increased incidence of circulating autoantibodies and overt autoimmune disease (*Figure 6.13*).

Immunology

Serum and secretory IgA are absent, but secretory component, a product of intestinal epithelial cells rather than plasma cells, is present in normal amounts. The antibody response to systemic immunization and studies of cell-mediated immunity are normal.

Pathogenesis

Selective IgA deficiency may have a wide range of causes. In most cases, no pattern of inheritance is found but autosomal recessive or dominant modes of transmission have been recorded sometimes. Occasionally, IgA deficiency has been associated with chromosomal defects and ataxia telangiectasia. Rarely, IgA deficiency is secondary to drug therapy, for example phenytoin or D-penicillamine.

Most IgA-deficient patients have normal numbers of peripheral B cells, including cells with surface IgA. In some cases, these IgA B cells respond to *in-vitro* stimulation by synthesizing intracytoplasmic IgA in small amounts. It has therefore been argued that either the T cells of these patients fail to help IgA-bearing B lymphocytes to respond to antigen, or a suppressor T cell population selectively inhibits IgA production. The experimental data required to resolve these alternatives are conflicting.

Selective IgM deficiency

In contrast to IgA deficiency, an isolated lack of IgM with normal concentration of other immunoglobulin classes is rare. About 20% of patients described have been asymptomatic and several cases have been detected fortuitously in middle age. The principal problem in the remainder is infection: about 30% develop septicaemia and 20% meningitis.

Selective IgG subclass deficiency

There are several examples of varying combinations of deficiencies of the four subclasses of IgG. Selective deficiencies of IgG_2, IgG_3 and IgG_4 subclasses are easily missed because of the dominant contribution made by IgG_1 to the total serum IgG level, which may remain within the normal range.

Major antibody activity can reside in a particular subclass: for example, IgG_2 dominates the antibody response to pneumococcal polysaccharide antigens. Subclass deficiency can thus predispose the individual to recurrent bacterial infections.

Complications of antibody deficiency

Patients with antibody deficiency suffer from a variety of complications (*Figure 6.14*).

Chronic infection

Chronic sepsis of upper and lower respiratory tracts leads to chronic otitis media, sinusitis, bronchiectasis, pulmonary fibrosis and, ultimately, cor pulmonale. Some adults

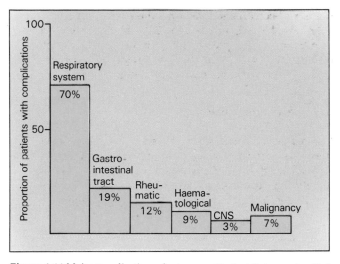

Figure 6.14 *Major complications of primary antibody deficiency, classified by organ involvement*

develop a granulomatous disease of the lungs resembling sarcoidosis. Although pyogenic bacteria cause most of the infective episodes some patients also show impaired handling of viruses. A few individuals, particularly those with the infantile sex-linked form of antibody deficiency, develop a rare but usually fatal dermatomyositis-like illness characterized by tense peripheral oedema, thickening of the skin and subcutaneous tissues, a violaceous skin rash, arthritis and meningoencephalitis. Echovirus has been consistently isolated from the CSF or brain.

Gastrointestinal disease

Mild gastrointestinal disease occurs in about two-thirds of adults with antibody deficiency and in one-quarter warrants further investigations.

Stomach

A pernicious anaemia-like syndrome is relatively common although it differs from classical pernicious anaemia in several ways: autoantibodies to parietal cells and intrinsic

factor are absent; the atrophic gastritis involves the whole stomach without antral sparing; and serum gastrin levels tend to be lower than in classical pernicious anaemia.

Small intestine

Mild malabsorption with diarrhoea occurs intermittently in over half of adults with hypogammaglobulinaemia. Bacterial overgrowth of the small intestine (commonly caused by *Campylobacter*) or infestation with *Giardia lamblia* or *Cryptosporidum* are responsible for most episodes. Jejunal biopsies show a spectrum of changes ranging from normality to subtotal villous atrophy. Villous regeneration may occur following antibiotics or immunoglobulin replacement therapy (so-called hypogammaglobulinaemic sprue): exceptionally, antibody deficiency may coexist with other intestinal disorders such as coeliac disease.

Hyperplasia of gut-associated lymphoid tissue occurs in some adults with common variable immunodeficiency, producing the radiological appearance of nodular lymphoid hyperplasia (NLH). Nodules can occur at any site in the gut, but typically affect the jejunum. This complication seems to occur in patients who have B lymphocytes and may represent a limited local immune response to antigen in the gut. NLH is benign but large nodules occasionally cause obstructive symptoms.

Liver

Chronic cholangitis caused by ascending bacterial infection of the biliary tracts is a recognized complication of antibody deficiency. Some cases progress to hepatic cirrhosis.

Rheumatic disease

An arthropathy complicates 10% of cases of antibody deficiency. Septic arthritis, and particularly *Mycoplasma* infection, should be excluded in all cases: of the remainder, some patients develop a chronic polyarthritis of large joints which responds to immunoglobulin replacement, while a minority suffer from apparently typical rheumatoid disease with erosive arthritis and subcutaneous nodules, but lack circulating rheumatoid factor. It is not uncommon for patients with antibody defects to be misdiagnosed initially as Still's disease or rheumatoid arthritis.

Other systemic complications

In spite of the absence of conventional antibodies, Coombs-positive haemolytic anaemia, autoimmune neutropenia and autoimmune thrombocytopenia have all been described.

Malignant disease

There is some evidence that patients with immunodeficiency states, either humoral or cell-mediated, have an increased incidence of malignant disease compared with

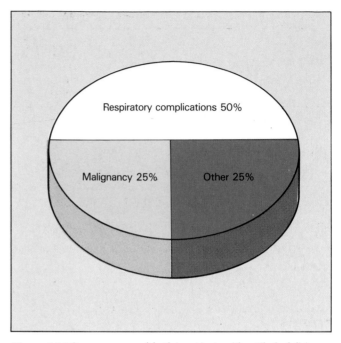

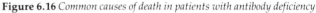

Figure 6.16 *Common causes of death in patients with antibody deficiency*

the general population. Malignancy has been reported in up to 15% of patients with certain types of immunodeficiency (*Table 6.2*), most tumours being of lymphoreticular origin (*Figure 6.15*).

However, the methods used in some of these studies are subject to statistical bias and the conclusions open to criticism. In some cases, the tumour has been the cause rather than the result of immunodeficiency.

Causes of death

Chronic respiratory disease and its complications account for approximately half of all deaths in patients with antibody deficiency (*Figure 6.16*). Unfortunately, many patients already have evidence of chronic lung damage by the time the diagnosis is made. Remaining causes of death vary between different series.

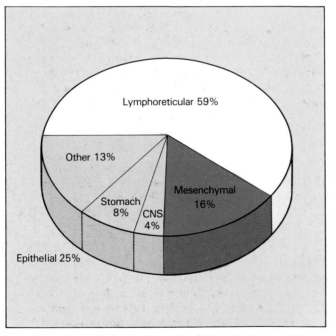

Figure 6.15 *Malignancy in patients with immunodeficiency, according to cell type*

Table 6.2 Malignancy in patients with primary immunodeficiency

Type of immunodeficiency	Patients who develop malignancy (per cent)	Mean age of patient at appearance of malignancy (years)
Selective IgA deficiency	2.5	30
Variable immunodeficiency		
Age at onset 0 to 15 years	2.5	46
Age at onset 16 + years	.8.5	
Infantile X-linked hypogammaglobulinaemia	0.7	8
Immunodeficiency with thrombocytopenia and eczema (Wiskott–Aldrich)	15	6
Ataxia telangiectasia	12	9

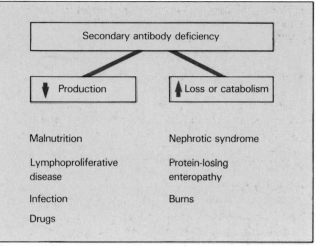

Figure 6.17 *Secondary causes of immunoglobulin deficiency*

Secondary causes of immunoglobulin deficiency

Secondary causes of immunoglobulin deficiency are far commoner than primary causes. In most cases, this is of minor relevance to the clinical picture but occasionally the severity of the immune defect may mask the underlying disease. Serum immunoglobulin levels represent the net balance of immunoglobulin synthesis versus immunoglobulin catabolism and loss, so low serum immunoglobulins reflect either grossly depressed production or increased loss and accelerated catabolism (*Figure 6.17*).

Impaired immunoglobulin synthesis

Protein-calorie malnutrition

Protein deficiency causes profound changes in many organs, including the immune system. Malnourished populations have an increased incidence of infectious disease with its resulting morbidity and mortality. The association is complex, because low-grade infection may hinder the nutrition of already severely malnourished people further. Reports of total serum immunoglobulin levels are conflicting: while it is probable that levels are normal or only marginally reduced, numerous studies have shown impaired specific antibody production following immunization with bacterial, viral or other antigens. Protein-calorie malnutrition is associated with even more striking defects in cell-mediated immunity, phagocyte function and complement activity. Many of these defects appear to be reversible following adequate protein and calorie supplementation of the diet.

Lymphoproliferative diseases

The frequency of opportunistic infections in patients with disseminated malignancy suggests an underlying immune defect but it is often difficult to distinguish between the immunosuppressive effects of the disease and those of the treatment.

Chronic lymphatic leukaemia

CLL is commonly associated with hypogammaglobulinaemia and recurrent chest infections which tend to become more severe as the disease progresses. IgM is usually the first class of immunoglobulin to be affected. In some cases, replacement immunoglobulin provides partial protection.

Acute leukaemia and non-Hodgkin's lymphoma

These may be associated with defects of both humoral and cell-mediated immunity but the severity of the primary condition usually overrides the clinical importance of such defects.

Hodgkin's disease

This is usually associated with significant impairment of cell-mediated immunity. In contrast, normal serum immunoglobulin levels are maintained until late in the disease.

Multiple myeloma

Most myeloma patients have depressed levels of normal (that is nonparaprotein) immunoglobulins but the level of the characteristic monoclonal immunoglobulin is raised.

Infections

In several infectious states, the microorganism paradoxically suppresses rather than stimulates the immune system. Transient impairment of cell-mediated immunity has been noted in viral illnesses, particularly measles, rubella, infectious mononucleosis and viral hepatitis, and in bacterial infections such as tuberculosis, brucellosis, leprosy and syphilis. In contrast, secondary infections occurring in patients with malaria and trypanosomiasis may be caused by defective antibody production but the mechanism is unclear.

Drugs

Immunosuppressive drugs affect many aspects of cell function and may impair lymphocyte and polymorph activity although severe hypogammaglobulinaemia is unusual. Patients receiving therapy for malignant disease or to prevent organ transplant rejection commonly develop unusual opportunistic infections.

Congenital disorders

Down's syndrome is associated with an increased incidence of infections, especially of the respiratory tract. Although serum immunoglobulin levels may be raised, specific antibody production is probably defective, as is cell-mediated immunity and polymorph function.

Increased loss of immunoglobulins

Protein loss severe enough to cause hypogammaglobulinaemia and hypoproteinaemia occurs mainly via the kidney in the nephrotic syndrome or through the gut in protein-losing enteropathy.

Nephrotic syndrome

The primary diagnosis usually presents little difficulty. Renal loss of immunoglobulin is at least partially selective so that IgM levels are maintained in spite of the fall in serum IgG.

Protein-losing enteropathy

Protein may be lost from the gut in a variety of inflammatory diseases including Crohn's disease, ulcerative colitis and coeliac disease. In intestinal lymphangiectasia (*Figure 6.18*), the dilated lymphatics leak both lymphocytes and protein. Affected individuals often have a severe hypogammaglobulinaemia, mainly involving IgG, and grossly impaired cell-mediated immunity. The patient may present with recurrent or unusual infections with minimal intestinal symptoms.

Hypercatabolism of immunoglobulins

A primary hypercatabolic state, as opposed to loss from the kidneys or gut, is rare. The diagnosis depends on demonstrating a reduced half-life of injected ^{125}I-labelled immunoglobulin in the absence of protein loss from the renal or gastrointestinal tracts. This occurs in dystrophia myotonica although such patients rarely experience recurrent infections.

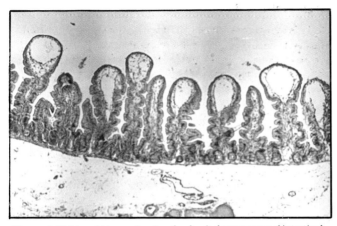

Figure 6.18 *Jejunal biopsy showing the classical appearance of intestinal lymphangiectasia: cyst-like, dilated central lacteals within the lamina propria of the villi. This patient, a 46-year-old female, presented with disseminated chicken pox*

Treatment of antibody deficiency states

Early recognition and diagnosis is essential to the successful management of those with defective immunity.

Immunoglobulin replacement

The major requirement of immunoglobulin replacement therapy is to give enough to prevent further infections and so reduce the incidence of complications.

Immunoglobulin injections

The standard immunoglobulin available for replacement therapy in the UK is prepared from out-dated pooled blood-bank plasma. Most of the material in this preparation is IgG at a concentration of about 150 g/l (approximately 15 times more concentrated than serum IgG). It also contains small amounts of other plasma proteins. The antibody activity of the preparation reflects the specificities of the donor pool.

Glycine is added as a stabilizer and thiomersal as a preservative. It remains stable for at least 4 years, provided that it is stored at +4°C to limit the formation of aggregates and has a half-life similar to that of native IgG (18–22 days). This immunoglobulin preparation is for intramuscular use only and must never be given intravenously because of the risk of inducing an acute vasomotor reaction.

The dose of immunoglobulin is related to the weight of the patient. A Medical Research Council trial compared the frequency of infection in patients receiving high (50 mg IgG/kg body weight), medium (25 mg IgG/kg) and low (12.5 mg IgG/kg) doses of immunoglobulin for the treatment of hypogammaglobulinaemia. The low dose was discontinued early in the trial because it appeared to be ineffective. Patients who received the medium or high dose had significantly fewer febrile episodes although some patients fared better on the high dose. Current practice in this country is based on that trial. Newly diagnosed patients are given loading doses of 50 mg IgG/kg body weight daily for 5 days, followed by 25 mg/kg/week thereafter. As a rough guide, most patients remain reasonably free from infections provided that the serum IgG level is maintained above 2 g/l. If infections persist, however, the dose can be increased to 50 mg/kg/week. If the clinical response to this raised dose is still unsatisfactory, then plasma infusions or intravenous immunoglobulin preparations may be of benefit.

Reactions to intramuscular immunoglobulin

Unfortunately, there are drawbacks to the use of the standard preparation (*Figure 6.19*). The most serious problem is that up to 20% of all patients will develop a systemic vasomotor reaction: these are usually isolated episodes and persist in only 2–4% of patients. The reactions generally occur within minutes of the injection and resemble classical anaphylactic reactions. Symptoms include pain in the limbs or back, faintness, breathlessness, fear of impending death and anxiety, accompanied by hypotension, loss of consciousness and fever. Rarely, deaths have occurred. The treatment of a reaction requires general measures for shock, and subcutaneous adrenaline and intravenous hydrocortisone should be available.

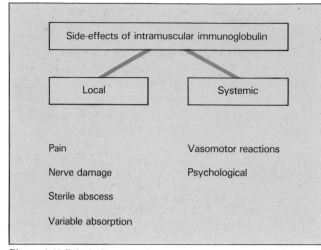

Figure 6.19 *Principal reactions to intramuscular immunoglobulin injections*

Most reactions occur sporadically and are almost certainly caused by aggregates of IgG in the preparation which activate complement and release vasoactive amines. As all preparations contain some aggregates, the relative rarity of reactions is probably caused by delayed absorption of aggregates following intramuscular injection and their elimination by phagocytes. Reactions are almost inevitable if the preparation is injected intravenously, suggesting that some of the reactions to intramuscular immunoglobulins are caused by part of the dose entering a vein.

The other major drawback is that the injections are painful. In an adult weighing 50 kg, the standard dose of 25 mg/kg requires a weekly injection volume of 8 ml. The addition of 1% lignocaine to the immunoglobulin may help most patients. In some cases, however, the pain and fear of further injections may necessitate switching the patient to alternative treatment.

The development of 'aggregate-free' immunoglobulin which can be injected intravenously is desirable. Although a number of such preparations are becoming commercially available, the advantages claimed for these intravenous immunoglobulins in terms of effectiveness, patient preference and a lower incidence of side effects must be balanced against the cost of long-term maintenance therapy.

Plasma infusions

Infusions of fresh plasma have several advantages over intramuscular immunoglobulin injections (*Figure 6.20*). At a dose of 10–15 ml of plasma per kilogram body weight every 2–3 weeks, IgG levels can be reached which are similar to those achieved by the conventional intramuscular regime. The advantages of the relatively painless volume that can be given must be weighed against the organizational problems of finding a suitable donor. Blood-bank plasma is not ideal because the risk of transmitting disease cannot be eliminated entirely. Plasma from a related donor can be used instead: selective immunization of this donor would provide the patient with specific passive immunity as required.

Plasma infusions are of benefit to those individuals who have frequent or severe reactions to immunoglobulin injections and those unable to accept the pain of this preparation.

Patients with selective IgA deficiency should not be treated with either intramuscular immunoglobulin or plasma infusion as they may produce high titres of anti-IgA antibodies.

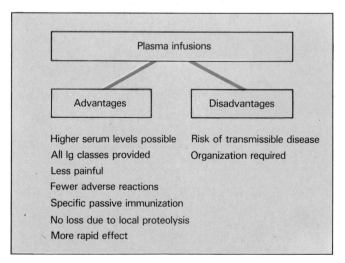

Figure 6.20 *Advantages and disadvantages of plasma infusions compared with intramuscular immunoglobulin injections*

General measures

Antibiotics

Although antibiotics should be started as soon as possible in the course of an infection, every effort must be made to identify the causative organism. Antibody-deficient patients respond as promptly as other patients to appropriate antibiotics but it is usually desirable to give at least 10 days' treatment. Long-term prophylactic antibiotics should be avoided as these encourage the growth of resistant organisms. However, some patients with bronchiectasis may require rotation of antibiotic therapy in addition to postural drainage. It should be emphasized that coexistent problems may be attributed mistakenly to the complications of hypogammaglobulinaemia: for example, an inhaled foreign body may be overlooked in the hypogammaglobulinaemic child with recurrent chest infections.

Immunization

Some antibody-deficient patients have developed untoward reactions following immunization with living attenuated organisms, for example poliovirus. It is therefore prudent to avoid 'live' vaccines in patients with suspected or proven defects in antibody production. Killed bacterial vaccines are generally harmless, although endotoxic shock has been described in some individuals following typhoid, paratyphoid A and paratyphoid B vaccination. In those patients who are receiving replacement immunoglobulin therapy, the passive immunity provided by the preparation considerably reduces the risk of contracting endemic infection.

Further reading

ASHERSON, G. L. and WEBSTER, A. D. B. (1980) *Diagnosis and Treatment of Immunodeficiency Diseases.* Blackwell, London

BUCKLEY, R. II. (1977) Replacement therapy in immunodeficiency. In *Recent Advances in Clinical Immunology*, vol. 1 (R. A. Thompson, ed.). Churchill Livingstone, Edinburgh

CHANDRA, R. K. (1980) Immunology of nutritional disorders. In *Current Topics in Immunology Series*, no. 12 (J. Turk, ed.). Arnold, London

CHANDRA, R. K. (1983) Trace elements and immune responses. *Immunology Today*, **4**, 322–325

HAYWARD, A. R. (1977) Immunodeficiency. In *Current Topics in Immunology Series*, no. 6 (J. Turk, ed.). Arnold, London

MEDICAL RESEARCH COUNCIL (1970) *Report SRS 310.* HMSO, London

THOMPSON, R. A. and REES-JONES, A. (1979) The antibody deficiency syndrome: a report on current management. *Journal of Infection*, **1**, 49

7 Defects of cell-mediated immunity

Defects of specific immunity can be classified into: (1) antibody deficiency, (2) selective impairment of cell-mediated immunity, and (3) combined deficiencies of cell-mediated immunity and antibody production.

Antibody deficiency is discussed in Chapter 6. Diseases caused by defective cell-mediated immunity are discussed in this chapter.

The assessment of cell-mediated immunity

Many assays of cellular immunity have been described. They vary considerably in complexity, specificity and availability. The following tests are in widespread usage by specialized immunology laboratories. However, early consultation between the clinician and the laboratory is essential if the assays are to be used judiciously.

Delayed hypersensitivity skin reactions

Recall antigens

Skin testing assumes that the patient has been sensitized previously to the test antigen. This assumption is more likely to be valid if a panel of four or five antigens is used: usually this will include purified protein derivative (PPD), *Candida albicans*, trichophytin, streptokinase–streptodornase (SK–SD) or mumps antigens, plus control solutions. Results should be read after 48 h and the diameter of erythema and induration recorded (*Figure 7.1*).

While 90% or more of healthy adults respond to at least one antigen from this panel, delayed hypersensitivity to recall antigens will be absent in infants or young children never previously exposed to the relevant pathogens. Since primary defects of cell-mediated immunity present mainly in this age group, an alternative method of judging skin reactivity is needed.

Active sensitization

Contact sensitizing agents, such as dinitrochlorobenzene (DNCB), can be used to sensitize deliberately patients lacking positive skin tests to recall antigens. A solution of DNCB in acetone is first carefully painted onto the skin and the patient challenged 10 days later with a more dilute solution of DNCB: normal individuals develop erythema and induration at the test site within 48 h. Care must be taken to avoid sensitization of staff handling this chemical.

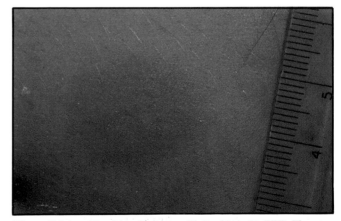

Figure 7.1 *A positive delayed hypersensitivity skin test to PPD. The antigen had been injected intradermally 48 h previously*

Total lymphocyte count

A lymphocyte count below 1×10^9 per litre in children is a useful screening test for some cellular defects, because many patients with severe combined immunodeficiency and some with thymic hypoplasia show persistent lymphopenia.

T-lymphocyte numbers

Circulating T cells can be counted by two methods: the simplest and most widely available is the sheep erythrocyte (E) rosette test. For reasons that are not clear, human T cells bind sheep red cells to form rosettes (*Figure 7.2*). About 60–80% of normal peripheral blood lymphocytes are T cells by this definition. Recently, a series of monoclonal antibodies has been raised in mice which recognizes T cells and their subsets. The monoclonal antibody will bind to the surface of any viable human cells expressing the appropriate antigen. Antibody-coated cells can then be stained with a fluorescein-labelled antibody to mouse immunoglobulin.

T-lymphocyte subsets

Monoclonal antisera also can distinguish thymocytes from peripheral T lymphocytes and helper from suppressor T cells. In normal blood, about 65% of T cells are helper cells and 35% are suppressor cells. Changes in these proportions may prove to be significant in the pathogenesis of some immunodeficiency diseases.

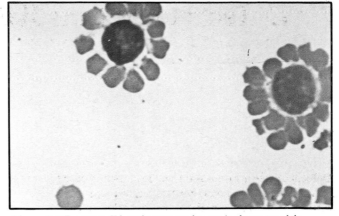

Figure 7.2 *E rosettes: T lymphocytes can be seen in the centre of the rosettes, surrounded by a layer of sheep red cells*

Lymphocyte transformation

Following stimulation, a few small, resting lymphocytes enlarge and change into blast cells showing DNA synthesis, a process termed lymphocyte transformation (*Figure 7.3*). Stimulating substances fall into three groups (*Table 7.1*).

When lymphocytes from two genetically different (i.e. allogeneic) people are mixed in cell culture, the T cells of each individual recognize and respond to histocompatibility antigens (*Figure 7.4*) presented by the cells of the other. This is called the mixed lymphocyte reaction (MLR). Donor cells can be stopped from transforming either by irradiation or by pretreatment with mitomycin, so any detectable

Table 7.1 Agents causing activation of T lymphocytes

Stimulating agent	Example	Specificity of response	Need for previous exposure	Degree of activation induced
Antigens	PPD	Specific	Yes	+
Mitogens	Phytohaemagglutinin	Nonspecific	No	+++
Allogeneic lymphocytes	Mixed lymphocyte reaction	Specific	No	++

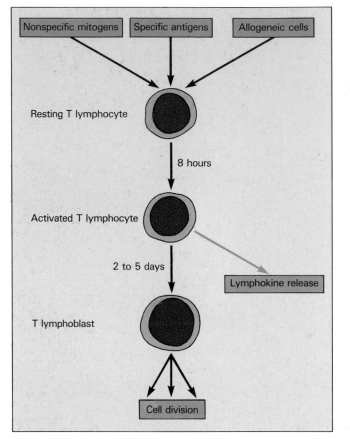

Figure 7.3 *Activation of T lymphocytes. T-cell function can be assessed readily either by measuring lymphokine production or by the degree of blast transformation following stimulation*

lymphocyte stimulation represents the response of the test lymphocytes to the allogeneic cells (a 'one-way' MLR). The MLR is a vital test in matching donor and recipient prior to bone-marrow transplantation.

Lymphokine release

Lymphocytes, when re-exposed to an antigen *in vitro*, release a variety of biologically active substances into the culture medium (*Figure 7.3*). These products of activated lymphocytes, called lymphokines, are regarded as possible mediators of delayed hypersensitivity reactions. One such lymphokine is leucocyte migration inhibition factor (LIF). The spontaneous migration, *in vitro*, of leucocytes from sensitized donors is inhibited specifically in the presence of an antigen to which the donor has been sensitized (*Figure 7.5*). This inhibition correlates with cell-mediated immunity but not with humoral immunity. It is known that polymorphs are the target cells, whereas lymphocytes are the effector cells, releasing the lymphokines that inhibit polymorph movement.

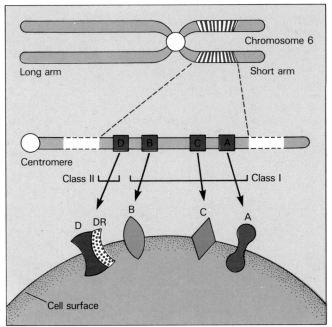

Figure 7.4 *The major histocompatibility complex in man, designated HLA, is situated on chromosome 6. The A and B loci code for serologically defined major transplantation antigens (Class I antigens) present on all cells (except erythrocytes) and for the target antigens with which cytotoxic T cells react. The DR region contains the serologically defined DR antigens (Class II antigens) present only on some cells, principally macrophages, B cells and activated T cells. DR antigens determine the magnitude of humoral responses to thymus-dependent antigens via their role in antigen presentation and helper T cell–B cell interaction. The MHC includes genes that code for certain components (C2, C4, factor B) of the complement system (Class III antigens)*

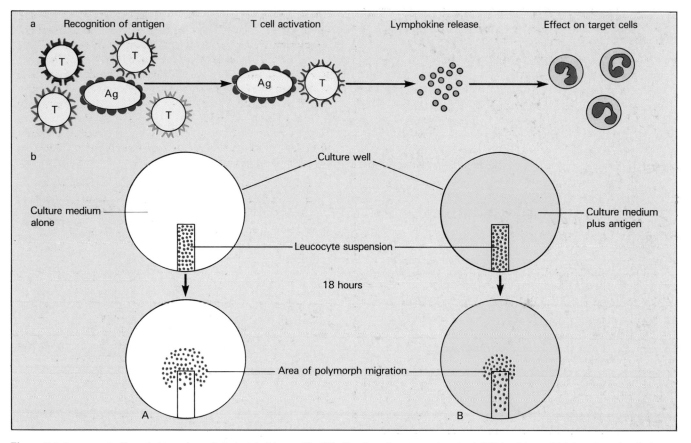

Figure 7.5 *Assessment of lymphokine release. In principle (a), sensitized T cells release leucocyte migration inhibition factor which impairs polymorph migration. In practice (b), the migration of leucocytes from capillary tubes is measured with and without antigen in the surrounding culture medium. Lymphokine release causes marked reduction in the area of polymorph migration. If the ratio of the area B ÷ area A is less than 0.8, it usually indicates that T cells in the leucocyte suspension were presensitized to the test antigen*

Other assays

Some patients with defective cell-mediated immunity lack the enzymes adenosine deaminase or purine nucleoside phosphorylase. These enzymes can be measured in lysates of red cells.

Selective defects of cell-mediated immunity

Isolated defects of T-cell function are rare. Usually, depressed T-cell immunity is accompanied by abnormalities of B-cell function, reflecting the degree of T–B cooperation necessary for antibody production to most antigens.

Thymic hypoplasia (Di George syndrome)

Pathogenesis

The thymus develops as an epithelial outgrowth of the third and fourth pharyngeal pouches at around the 8th to 12th weeks of embryonic life. The parathyroid glands and parts of the primitive aortic arch are derived from the same regions. The complete form of the Di George syndrome (*Figure 7.6*) is thus characterized by cardiovascular abnormalities with parathyroid and thymic hypoplasia. The cause is unknown. There is usually no familial trend, so presumably the intrauterine damage is caused by an environmental agent such as a drug or a virus, but none has been identified.

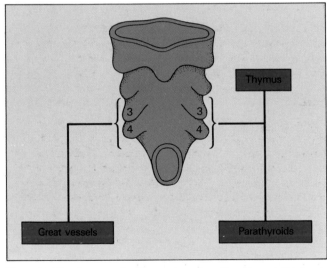

Figure 7.6 *Development of major structures from the embryonic third and fourth pharyngeal pouches*

Clinical features

The Di George syndrome is one of the few immunodeficiency disorders associated with symptoms shortly after birth. Severely affected infants present with hypocalcaemic convulsions, tetany or cardiovascular defects. Susceptibility to infection is variable. Most deaths in the neonatal period are due to the cardiac malformations. Patients who survive their cardiac problems long enough to develop infections suffer from pneumonia, diarrhoea and candidiasis.

In some infants, the diagnosis is suggested by an abnormal facial appearance of low-set malformed ears, hypertelorism, micrognathia and cleft palate.

Immunological features

Most patients have a raised proportion of B lymphocytes and a lowered percentage of T cells although lymphopenia is an inconstant finding. Lymphocyte transformation is poor or absent yet serum immunoglobulins and antibody responses to test immunization may be normal sometimes, which is surprising in view of the need for T cells in antibody production.

Some infants with this condition gradually but spontaneously develop cellular immunity without specific treatment, a subgroup termed 'partial Di George syndrome'.

The Di George syndrome is a potentially treatable condition: several infants have been grafted successfully with human fetal thymus (see below).

Purine nucleoside phosphorylase deficiency

Purine nucleoside phosphorylase (PNP) deficiency is an example of immunodeficiency caused by an inherited enzyme defect.

Pathogenesis

The condition is due to a defective structural gene coding for PNP on chromosome 14. PNP converts inosine and guanosine to their corresponding bases hypoxanthine and guanine (*Figure 7.7*). In PNP deficiency, high plasma and urinary levels of inosine, deoxyinosine, guanosine and deoxyguanosine occur, with correspondingly low plasma and urine uric acid concentrations. Deoxyguanosine triphosphate accumulates within lymphocytes and blocks DNA synthesis. T cells are affected more than B cells, although the biochemical reasons for this difference are not yet resolved entirely.

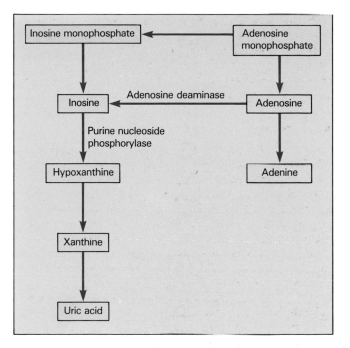

Figure 7.7 *Simplified diagram of the purine salvage pathways, showing the sites of action of PNP and ADA*

Chronic mucocutaneous candidiasis

Clinical features

Typically, there is chronic and often disfiguring *Candida albicans* infection of mucous membranes, nails and skin although the severity of the lesions may vary considerably. Associated endocrine abnormalities are frequent: idiopathic hypoparathyroidism is the most common lesion, followed by autoimmume adrenalitis (Addison's disease) and then a variety of disorders, including hypogonadism, diabetes mellitus, hypothyroidism, pernicious anaemia, vitiligo and alopecia. Many cases show a familial tendency.

Some years may elapse between the onset of the endocrine lesions and the onset of candidiasis.

Immunological features

Most patients make good antibody responses to Candida yet lack cell-mediated immunity to the organism. Lymphocyte responses to mitogens, to allogeneic cells and to antigens other than Candida are usually normal.

Treatment

Treatment is difficult. Antifungal agents, such as miconazole or amphoteracin B, usually will eradicate the candidiasis temporarily but most patients relapse and the toxicity of many antifungal drugs prevents their prolonged usage. Early reports suggest that ketoconazole will prove to be a safe and effective agent in this condition. The combination of antifungal drugs and transfer factor therapy (see below) may also be beneficial.

Combined immunodeficiency

In combined immunodeficiency, both humoral and cell-mediated immune mechanisms are defective.

Severe combined immunodeficiency

Severe combined immunodeficiency (SCID) includes a heterogeneous group of syndromes (*Table 2*).

Affected infants are susceptible to a wide spectrum of infections. Until recently, the condition was incurable and

Clinical features

Affected children have experienced recurrent upper and lower respiratory tract infections in the first year of life. Viruses, particularly varicella, cytomegalovirus and herpes, have also been handled abnormally and some patients additionally developed autoimmune haemolytic anaemia.

Immunological features

T-cell numbers are low, with impaired lymphocyte transformation responses and negative skin tests but these changes are not diagnostic. Serum immunoglobulin levels and specific antibody responses have been normal.

Plasma and urine uric acid levels are simple screening tests although definite diagnosis depends on measurement of PNP levels in lysates of red cells.

Table 7.2 Subgroups of severe combined immunodeficiency

1. SCID (Swiss-type)
2. SCID with ADA deficiency
3. SCID with B lymphocytes
4. Bare lymphocyte syndrome
5. Reticular dysgenesis

death was inevitable. In 1968, however, two teams successfully corrected SCID by bone marrow transplantation. Since then, this approach has been studied intensively as a treatment not only for SCID but also for disorders such as leukaemia and aplastic anaemia.

Clinical features

The commonest presentation is diarrhoea and failure to thrive: the condition is often suspected only after multiple episodes of 'gastroenteritis'. Mucocutaneous candidiasis and pneumonia, often due to opportunistic organisms such as *Candida albicans* or *Pneumocystis carinii*, are frequent.

In contrast to the antibody deficiency syndrome, all infants with SCID are symptomatic before the age of 6 months. Boys are affected twice as often as girls but there are few diagnostically useful physical signs.

Immunological features

Immunological diagnosis rests on the demonstration, firstly, of panhypogammaglobulinaemia with poor specific antibody production and, secondly, of defective cell-mediated immunity. Most infants also have significant lymphopenia, that is, absolute lymphocyte counts below 1×10^9 per litre. The diagnosis can be made before birth by examining fetal lymphocytes obtained at fetoscopy.

SCID associated with adenosine deaminase deficiency

Adenosine deaminase (ADA) deficiency accounts for about one-third of all cases of SCID.

Pathogenesis

ADA catalyses the conversion of adenosine or deoxyadenosine to inosine or deoxyinosine (*Figure 7.7*). In the absence of ADA, deoxyadenosine triphosphate accumulates within cells and blocks DNA synthesis. Lymphocytes, especially T cells, are affected selectively. The enzyme is present in most tissues of the body and can be measured conveniently in lysates of red blood cells.

ADA is the product of a gene carried on chromosome 20. Some families with SCID inherit a null gene which does not give rise to a detectable product. Homozygous inheritance of this null gene is responsible for SCID asociated with ADA deficiency. Parents and heterozygote siblings have roughly half-normal activity of red-cell ADA. Prenatal diagnosis is possible by measurement of ADA activity in amniotic fluid cells.

Clinical features

The clinical features are similar to those infants with SCID who have normal ADA activity. However, nonimmunological manifestations of ADA deficiency may also occur: these include defective bone ossification with flaring and cupping of the anterior ends of the ribs and growth arrest lines in the long bones.

Severely affected infants die within 1–2 years unless appropriately treated. Some infants are normal at birth because the mother's metabolic pathways remove accumulating deoxyadenosine, but these infants subsequently deteriorate.

Successful bone-marrow transplantation is curative but carries considerable risk (see below). Enzyme replacement is an alternative form of treatment and some ADA-deficient infants have improved after repeated transfusions of red cells (as a source of ADA) from healthy donors.

SCID with immunoglobulins

Some children with SCID differ from those with other forms in having normal serum levels of one or more immunoglobulin classes. However, their antibody responses to test immunizations remain depressed.

This subgroup has sometimes been called the Nezelof syndrome. This term is neither descriptive nor used consistently and probably is best abandoned.

The bare lymphocyte syndrome

The bare lymphocyte syndrome is characterized by combined immunodeficiency with failure to express HLA-A, -B and -C locus antigens and $\beta2$-microglobulin on lymphocytes.

Major clinical features include candidiasis, pneumonia, diarrhoea and failure to thrive. In some patients, T-cell functions are grossly abnormal; in others T-cells acquire proliferative activity to mitogens but not antigens and fail to cooperate with B cells in antibody production.

HLA-A, -B and -C antigens are composed of one α polypeptide chain joined to one β chain. The β chain apparently is identical with $\beta2$-microglobulin. As a result of the absence or reduction in surface $\beta2$-microglobulin, HLA antigens fail to anchor to cell membranes. Because HLR-DR antigens do not contain $\beta2$-microglobulin, their expression is not affected.

This syndrome highlights the importance of HLA molecules in the development of functional T lymphocytes.

SCID with leucopenia (reticular dysgenesis)

Affected infants have severe functional defects of granulocytes and lymphocytes. The cause of the defect is not yet known. Infections begin in the neonatal period and death follows within the first 3 months.

Ataxia telangiectasia

Ataxia telangiectasia is an inherited multisystem disorder, characterized by progressive neurological degeneration, oculocutaneous telangiectasia and immunodeficiency.

Pathogenesis

The underlying defect is unknown but may involve defective DNA repair since lymphocytes from affected patients have an increased sensitivity to low doses of

irradiation and to chemicals. Chromosome breaks have been found in about 25% of patients.

The disease is inherited in an autosomal recessive fashion.

Clinical features

Most cases present in childhood with difficulty in walking caused by cerebellar ataxia. The neurological disorder is progressive and ultimately leads to choreoathetosis, pyramidal tract signs and intellectual deterioration. The characteristic telangiectasia may not appear for some years after the neurological signs. They first occur on the exposed bulbar conjunctiva and later on the nose, ears and shoulders. Over 75% of patients experience recurrent respiratory tract infections.

The incidence of malignant disease in ataxia telangiectasis shows a striking increase: lymphoreticular or epithelial tumours occur in 10–15% of patients. Family members also have a high incidence of malignancy.

Immunological features

About three-quarters of patients have IgE and IgA deficiency. Although specific antibody is made, peak responses to test antigens are often subnormal. Cellular immunity may be depressed only mildly in younger patients but becomes progressively more abnormal as the children get older.

Raised serum α-fetoprotein levels are a useful diagnostic feature but not an indicator of malignancy.

Treatment

No treatment will halt the neurological deterioration of the condition. Although a number of approaches have been used to try to modify the immunodeficiency, it is doubtful whether these are justified until the neurological deterioration can first be arrested.

Wiskott-Aldrich syndrome

This disorder is characterized by thrombocytopenia, eczema and immunodeficiency. The condition is inherited as an X-linked recessive trait but the underlying cause is unknown.

Clinical features

Without effective treatment, the disease runs a fluctuating but progressive course, leading to death in infancy or early childhood. Occasionally, patients may survive to early adult life.

Platelet numbers are characteristically low. The platelets are small and fail to aggregate normally. Consequently, bleeding is often the most serious clinical problem: it may present as bloody diarrhoea or even intracerebral haemorrhage. The eczema has the distribution typical of atopic eczema and is prone to secondary infection.

Recurrent bacterial infections, such as pneumonia, otitis media, sinusitis, meningitis and staphylococcal skin sepsis are common, but viral infections are usually less troublesome.

Immunological features

The immunological findings are not diagnostic. Antibody responses to test immunizations are poor and there is a variable impairment of cell-mediated immunity. Affected individuals have an increased incidence of lymphoreticular malignancy.

It has been argued that the defects in the Wiskott-Aldrich syndrome result from impaired macrophage function, so that improperly processed antigen cannot stimulate T and B cells correctly: proof of this hypothesis is lacking.

Treatment

Treatment is required to control the bleeding tendency, recurrent infections, eczema and malignancy.

The thrombocytopenia is usually resistant both to steroids and to splenectomy. Splenectomy also carries the risk of subsequent fulminating septicaemia. The eczema may be of allergic origin since it is often accompanied by positive prick tests, eosinophilia and a high serum IgE. Where possible, allergens should be identified and avoided.

There is anecdotal evidence that the frequency of infections can be reduced and the platelet count improved by treatment with transfer factor (see below). However, the objective value of transfer factor is debatable. The poor prognosis of the Wiskott-Aldrich syndrome makes bone-marrow transplantation a justifiable procedure when a histocompatible sibling donor is available and some successful transplants have been claimed.

Secondary causes of impaired cell-mediated immunity

Secondary causes of immunodeficiency are far commoner than primary causes and are discussed in Chapter 6. Impaired cellular immunity accompanying malnutrition and parasitic, bacterial or viral infections is a major cause of morbidity for a large part of the world's population.

The recently-recognized *acquired immunodeficiency syndrome (AIDS)* may be caused by an immunosuppressive microorganism. The syndrome is characterized by the development of severe, disseminated opportunistic infections (particularly *Pneumocystis carinii* pneumonia) and Kaposi's sarcoma. About 75% of cases have occurred in previously healthy, young, homosexual American men, and about 40% of those affected have already died. Patients show cutaneous anergy, decreased lymphocyte transformation responses and striking lymphopenia; total T lymphocytes are profoundly reduced and the helper to suppressor T-cell ratio reversed because the helper-cell subpopulation is almost absent.

In an analysis of the risk factors in homosexuals, significant associations were found with multiple drug abuse and sexual promiscuity. Homosexual men, especially those who are indiscriminately promiscuous, are likely to contract a range of sexually transmitted diseases. Such homosexuals are often drug abusers and about 17% of the heterosexual victims of the syndrome have also been drug addicts. Many cases can be shown to have had direct sexual contact or to have shared intravenous needles used for 'mainlining' drugs. One per cent of cases occur in haemophiliacs and are believed to be related to their frequent intravenous injections of commercial factor VIII concentrates from the USA. About 5% of cases have occurred in individuals who do not fall into any of the known 'at risk' groups. As yet the unanswered question is the nature of the microorganism, but preliminary evidence suggests that a retrovirus with selective tropism for helper T cells is responsible for this devastating illness.

Therapeutic approaches to the treatment of impaired cell-mediated immunity

Early recognition is essential to the successful management of any patient with impaired immunity.

General measures

Genetic counselling

The prevention of primary immunodeficiency by genetic counselling is a feasible proposition for those conditions with a known mode of inheritance. However, caution must be exercised in assuming the pattern of inheritance in any family with only one affected member.

In a limited number of disorders, carriers of the abnormal genes can be identified.

Prenatal diagnosis

Once a biochemical defect has been defined, prenatal diagnosis becomes possible. For example, in ADA deficiency, prenatal prediction of affected babies can be made by measurement of ADA activity in cultured amniotic fluid fibroblasts obtained at amniocentesis. Identification of the sex of the fetus may also be helpful in families with a history of sex-linked immunodeficiencies.

Immunizations

Immunization with live vaccines, for example BCG, should be avoided in patients in whom impaired cellular immunity is suspected.

Avoidance of blood transfusions

Conventional blood transfusions must never be given to patients with proven or suspected defects in cell-mediated immunity because transfused donor T-lymphocytes may cause fatal graft-versus-host disease (GVHD) (see below). T cells remain viable for several weeks, not only in whole blood but also in washed red-cell, plasma and platelet preparations. If transfusion is necessary, the graft-versus-host potential of the blood must be eradicated either by irradiation (3000 rad) or by using deep-frozen, thawed and washed erythrocytes.

Antimicrobial therapy

Only complete environmental protection from birth, in either a totally enclosed atmosphere or a laminar flow room, can avoid effectively all infection. The practical and psychological problems of this approach are immense. In the more usual case, diagnosed after infections have occurred, full doses of the appropriate antibiotics should be commenced early after sensitivity testing of the micro-organisms.

Permanent grafting of immunocompetent tissues

Grafting of viable immunocompetent cells offers the only hope of permanent restoration of immune responsiveness yet carries with it the considerable dangers of inducing GVHD.

Bone-marrow transplantation

Donor selection

Transplantation of bone-marrow cells has been successful in many children with severe combined immunodeficiency. Donor and recipient should be HLA-identical. This requirement is of critical importance and usually met only by siblings. A person's histocompatibility antigens (tissue-type) are inherited as a series of closely linked genes (the HLA-haplotype) on a segment of chromosome 6 (*Figure 7.4*). Because one haplotype is inherited from each parent,

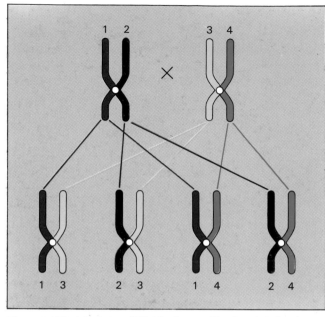

Figure 7.8 *The inheritance of HLA haplotypes. Numbers 1, 2, 3 and 4 refer to the complete HLA haplotypes of the parents. There is a one in four chance that two offspring will inherit identical haplotypes*

there is only a one-in-four chance that two siblings will have identical pairs of haplotypes (*Figure 7.8*). The trend towards small families limits the number of cases for whom there is a suitable sibling donor and in these patients bone-marrow transplantation has been attempted using mismatched marrow. Results of marrow transplantation (*Figure 7.9*) clearly show that transplants from HLA-D-locus-incompatible donors (as defined by a positive MLR) invariably fail, with all recipients developing GVHD and severe infections leading to death. It has been recommended therefore that HLA-D-locus-mismatched-marrow transplantation for SCID should be abandoned.

Successful transplantation has been achieved with marrow from matched but unrelated donors: special attention must be paid to the result of the MLR. In the first patient successfully engrafted with marrow from an unrelated but HLA-D-locus-compatible donor, reconstitu-

tion was achieved only after seven grafts and transplantation of 100 times more than the usual cell numbers.

Transplantation of cells

The actual procedure of bone-marrow transplantation is simple. Small amounts of bone marrow are taken from multiple sites under general anaesthesia. Bony spicules are

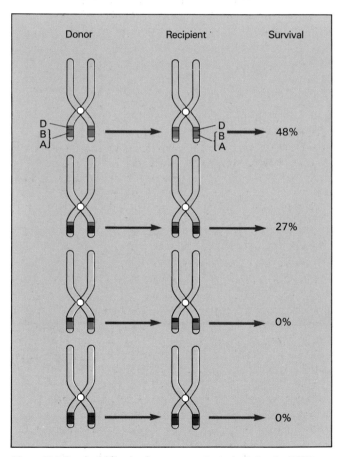

Figure 7.9 *Survival following bone-marrow transplantation for SCID. Survival is best when donor and recipient are both HLA and MLR matched. Mismatching at the D locus (MLR mismatched) is particularly associated with poor survival (matched = green, mismatched = red)*

removed by filtration through graded sets of sieves. Cells can be administered then without fractionation or subjected to methods intended to remove the cells causing GVHD. Transplanted cells are given by intravenous infusion or occasionally, in very small children, by intraperitoneal injection.

The optimal size of the graft is probably between 1 and 3×10^8 nucleated bone-marrow cells per kilogram body weight. Engraftment is unlikely with fewer than 1×10^7 cells per kilogram while greater than 3×10^8 cells per kilogram may be associated with severe GVHD.

Complications of transplantation: problems of GVHD

Three major complications dominate the post-transplant period: failure of the graft to 'take', GVHD and infection. Failure of engraftment can be due to using too few bone-marrow cells or to other factors as yet unknown. Manoeuvres to prevent and treat infection include nursing in strict, reverse isolation, skin and gut decontamination, gammaglobulin injections and appropriate antibiotics and antimycotics, although the need for all such measures is debatable. About 80% of deaths occur within 4 months of transplantation: the commonest cause is infection, one-third being due to *Pneumocystis carinii* pneumonia. Prophylactic treatment of Pneumocystis before and after transplantation therefore has been recommended.

If the grafted cells do survive and become established, their immunological activity may be directed against their new environment (*Figure 7.10*). GVHD appears 1–2 weeks after transplantation (or blood transfusion) and is characterized (*Figure 7.11*) by fever, an erythematous maculopapular rash, bloody diarrhoea, hepatitis, splenomegaly, aplastic or haemolytic anaemia, pulmonary infiltration, weight loss and death.

Prevention and elimination of GVHD has met with varied success. The most important single factor is undoubtedly histocompatibility. Once established, severe GVHD has never been treated with convincing and consistent effectiveness. Efforts have been directed therefore towards the elimination or reduction of the numbers of immunocompetent T cells (responsible for GVHD) in the graft. To date, such efforts have been disappointing:

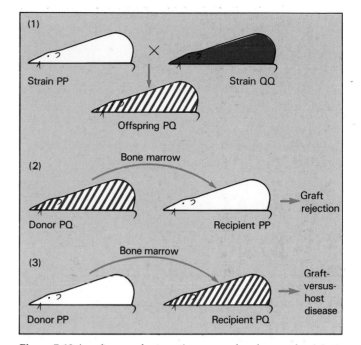

Figure 7.10 *A graft-versus-host reaction occurs when donor and recipient cells are histoincompatible and the immunocompetent lymphoid cells in the graft try to reject the host. Graft-versus-host reactions can be induced readily in animals genetically unable to reject grafted cells. This is achieved by transfer of cells from the parent (PP) to the first generation offspring (PQ) which is naturally tolerant of the parental antigens (P). However, the other set of parental antigens (Q) in the offspring are recognized as foreign by the grafted cells which mount a graft-versus-host reaction*

procedures currently being tested include the use of cyclosporin A to suppress the GVHD and pre-incubation of marrow with monoclonal antibodies or plant lectins to remove the T-cell subpopulations responsible for graft-versus-host responses. GVHD is more severe in boys who receive marrow from a sister, probably because of the distinctive antigens carried by male cells. Therefore, brothers are best used as marrow donors for boys with SCID.

The prognosis is improved if marrow transplantation is performed before the recipient is 6 months old: GVHD is more severe in older infants.

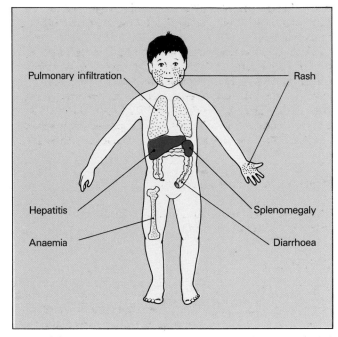

Figure 7.11 *Major clinical features of GVHD in man*

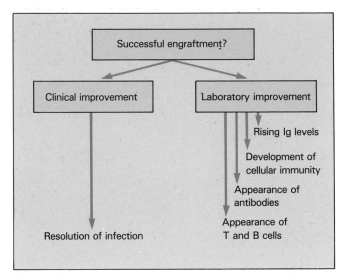

Figure 7.12 *Indirect evidence that successful bone-marrow engraftment has occurred*

Evidence of engraftment

Donor and recipient are usually studied before transplantation to find markers capable of showing whether or not engraftment has occurred, since failure of a graft to 'take' is an indication for repeating the transplant with a larger number of cells. Such markers include the X chromosome (if donor and recipient are of opposite sex), red cell antigens, immunoglobulin allotypes and enzyme activity in ADA-deficient patients. Indirect evidence of a functioning graft is reflected by the restoration of immune competence (*Figure 7.12*).

Other tissues

An alternative approach to marrow transplantation stems from the hope that non-matched tissue, if of fetal origin, will become tolerant of the recipient's HLA antigens and

thus be less likely to trigger GVHD. Unfortunately, both fetal thymus and fetal liver cells have been responsible for fatal GVHD. However, some patients have been improved dramatically by fetal grafts. They fall into two main groups: those with SCID who received fetal liver grafts with or without fetal thymus and those with the Di George syndrome who have benefited from fetal thymus.

Fetal liver

Fetal liver is a source of stem cells. Haematopoiesis begins at a gestational age of 4 weeks. B-lymphocytes appear at the twelfth week and mitogen-responsive cells after 18 weeks. Fetal liver transplantation, sometimes in combination with the thymus of the *same* fetus, produces a slow immunological reconstitution with a mild-to-moderate degree of GVHD. The main difficulty with fetal liver grafts is in producing a 'take': in several patients, engraftment either has been too short-lived or has consisted mainly of T-cell function.

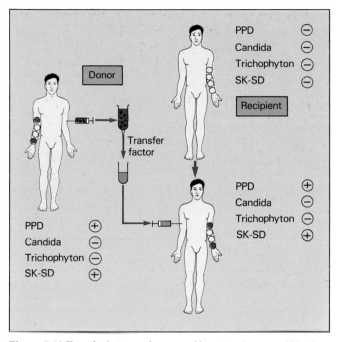

Figure 7.13 *Transfer factor can be prepared by extracting normal blood lymphocytes, dialysing the extract and freeze-drying the low-molecular-weight fraction. Subcutaneous injection of reconstituted transfer factor may transfer specific cellular immunity to the recipient. This is illustrated by the transfer of positive delayed hypersensitivity skin tests to purified protein derivative of* Mycobacterium tuberculosis *(PPD) and streptokinase–streptodornase (SK–SD)*

Fetal thymus

Fetal thymus contains not only T cells but also epithelial cells which are believed to produce hormonal factors influencing T-lymphocyte maturation. Transplantation of thymus from fetuses of 7–12 weeks' gestation has restored cell-mediated immunity in immunodeficient children, particularly those with thymic hypoplasia (Di George syndrome), and some suffering from chronic mucocutaneous candidiasis, ataxia telangiectasia or SCID. Following successful grafts, lymphocyte responsiveness to mitogens has improved within hours or days: the striking speed of this effect, and the observation, in at least one case, of improvement even when the thymus was enclosed

in a cell-impermeable millipore chamber suggest that hormonal factors released by the thymic epithelial cells are responsible.

More recently, thymic tissue obtained from children undergoing open-heart surgery has been cultered *in vitro* for about 3 weeks before transplantation. During this culture period lymphocytes disappear and with them, it is hoped, the capacity to induce GVHD. The epithelial cells remain. Cultured thymic epithelium reportedly has reconstituted both T- and B-cell function in patients with SCID.

Replacement of missing factors

The replacement of putative missing factors has met with varying degrees of success.

Cell extracts

Thymic factors

A range of thymic extracts has been prepared in recent years. In spite of some encouraging early results in the treatment of primary immunodeficiency, these preparations seem to be of limited usefulness. In general, often it has been easier to obtain increased numbers of E-rosetting cells in the laboratory than to confer significant benefit on the patient. It is likely that the different preparations available have different biological effects. As yet, it is not known which patients are likely to benefit, nor is the correct dose or route of administration known for each of the various preparations.

Transfer factor

Transfer factor is a low-molecular-weight, dialysable extract from normal blood lymphocytes which confers specific immune reactivity from a sensitive donor to a previously unsensitized individual. Only the spectrum of reactivity possessed by the donor lymphocytes is transferable (*Figure 7.13*).

Transfer factor (or dialysable leucocyte extract) has induced clinical and laboratory improvement in patients with the Wiskott-Aldrich syndrome, chronic mucocutaneous candidiasis and immunodeficiency secondary to leukaemia. However, this effect has not been confirmed by other workers and transfer factor has been the subject of considerable debate, particularly with respect to its apparant specificity, mode of action, clinical efficacy and even its very existence as a discrete entity.

Enzyme replacement

Erythrocytes contain ADA: frozen, irradiated red blood cells provide a source of this enzyme and hence effective treatment for some infants with SCID associated with ADA deficiency. One limitation of this approach is the need for repeated transfusions at monthly intervals.

Conclusion

During the past 15 years, knowledge of the normal immune response has expanded rapidly as a result of experimental work in animals and the study of primary immunodeficiency diseases in man. An outstanding example is seen in the consequences of genetic and biochemical defects of enzymes of the purine salvage pathways that are expressed mainly as immunodeficiency diseases.

Further reading

ASHERSON, G. L. and WEBSTER, A. D. B. (1980) *Diagnosis and Treatment of Immunodeficiency Diseases*. Blackwell, Oxford

BUCKLEY, R. H. (1977) Replacement therapy in immunodeficiency. In *Recent Advances in Clinical Immunology*, No. 1. (R. A. Thompson, ed.). Churchill Livingstone, Edinburgh

DENMAN, A. M. (1982) Graft-versus-host disease. *British Medical Journal*, **285**, 1226–1227

GIBSON, J., BASTEN, A. and VAN DER BRINK, C. (1983) Clinical use of transfer factor: 25 years on. *Clinics in Immunology and Allergy*, **3**, 331–357

HAYWARD, A. R. (1977) Immunodeficiency. In *Current Topics in Immunology Series*, No. 6. (J. Turk, ed.). Arnold, London

LEVINSKY, R. J. (1983) Marrow and thymus replacement in the repair of immunodeficiency *Clinics in Immunology and Allergy*, **3**, 207–228

KENNY, A. B. and HITZIG, W. H. (1979) Bone marrow transplantation for severe combined immunodeficiency disease. *European Journal of Paediatrics*, **131**, 155–177

PINCHING, A. (1984) The probable cause of AIDS. *Immunology Today*, **5**, 196–199

ROSENBLATT, H. M. and STIEHM, E. R. (1983) Therapy of chronic mucocutaneous candidiasis. *American Journal of Medicine*, **74**, 20–22

THORSBY, E. (1983) Structure and function of MHC. Power of molecular genetics amply confirmed. *Immunology Today*, **4**, 312–315

WORLD HEALTH ORGANIZATION (1979) Immunodeficiency. Report of a WHO Scientific Group. *Clinical Immunology and Immunopathy*, **13**, 296–359

8 Disorders of neutrophil function

Introduction

The major role of neutrophil leucocytes is to ingest, kill and digest invading microorganisms, particularly bacteria and fungi. Failure to fulfil this role leads to recurrent, severe or chronic infections, often with a family history of similar problems. Neutrophil activity can be subdivided conveniently into stages (*Figure 8.1*) and qualitative defects classified according to the functional step affected.

Normal neutrophil function (*Figure 8.1*)

Development and circulation

Neutrophils are produced in the bone marrow from white-cell precursors which are in turn derived from pluripotential stem cells. Initial stages, from stem cells through to myeloblasts, promyelocytes and myelocytes, involve three to five cell divisions over about 7 days. The neutrophil myeloid precursors then mature through nondividing stages of metamyelocytes and segmented forms over the next week to form a storage pool of matured cells.

Within the marrow, the precursor pool of mitotic cells and the storage pool together comprise about 94% of all neutrophils, considerably outnumbering neutrophil numbers in blood (*Figure 8.2*). Approximately 1.5×10^9 neutrophils per kilogram body weight are released into the circulation daily, where they are distributed equally between a population which circulates freely and a marginated pool which lies along the endothelial surfaces of small blood vessels. In bacterial infections, more cells enter the marginated pool and migrate into tissues under the influence of chemical attractants. This shift is usually balanced by a release of neutrophils from the marrow reserve pool. Normally, neutrophils spend only about 12 h in the circulation before entering the tissues, where they remain for 2–4 days.

In neutropenic individuals, it can be useful to know whether cells in the marrow reserve pool can be induced to move into the circulation or whether circulating cells have been depleted by margination. Provocation with intravenous hydrocortisone should cause marrow cells to enter the circulation, with a subsequent rise in the circulating neutrophil count of greater than 50% some 2–6 h later. Subcutaneous adrenaline or endotoxin will cause marginated cells to be detached from the marginated into the circulating pool; normally the neutrophil count will rise by more than 45% in 1 h.

Adhesion

Neutrophils must adhere first to the endothelial lining of the vessel wall before they can get out of the vessel. Within minutes of tissue damage or microbial invasion, marginated neutrophils adhere to the vessel wall, project pseudopodia between the vascular endothelial cells and then migrate into the surrounding tissues.

Movement

Accumulation of neutrophils at an inflammatory focus is enhanced by the ability of the neutrophil to migrate along a

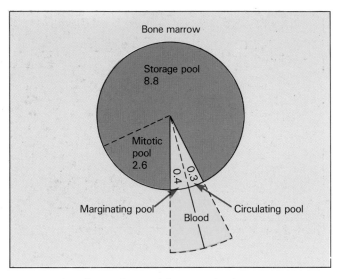

Figure 8.2 *Distribution of neutrophils in normal individuals. Figures show numbers of cells $\times 10^9$ per kilogram body weight*

concentration gradient of a chemoattractant, an effect termed chemotaxis. Potent chemotactic factors are generated via immunological and nonimmunological pathways (*Figure 8.3*).

Neutrophils posses contractile microfilaments composed of actin and myosin. Binding of chemotactic factors by specific receptors on the neutrophil cell membrane causes polymerization of actin and its assembly into microfilaments. Microtubules formed throughout the cell probably supply the structural framework needed for movement.

Measurement of neutrophil movement

One method of assessment is to produce an inflammatory focus and measure the rate at which neutrophils arrive at this site. In the Rebuck 'skin window' technique, skin of the forearm is abraded and the cells collected on a superimposed coverslip. Chemotaxis *in vitro* is measured traditionally in a Boyden chamber (*Figure 8.4*) although alternative methods exist.

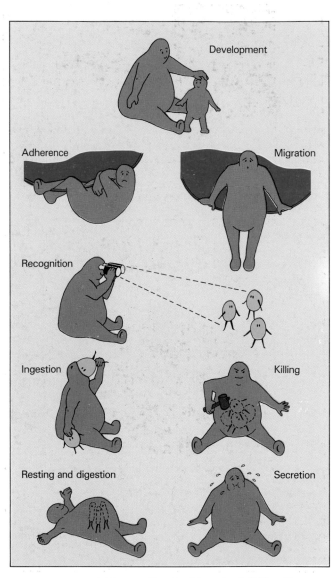

Figure 8.1 *Neutrophil function (Reprinted from Segal, 1980, with permission)*

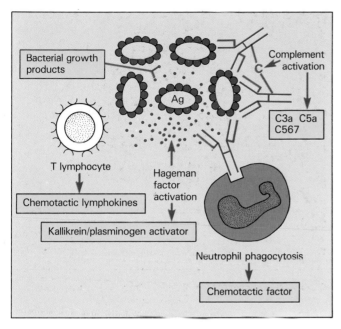

Figure 8.3 *Sources of chemotactic factors*

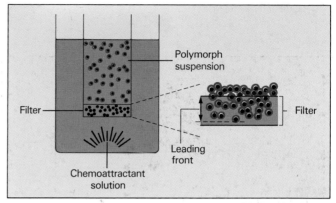

Figure 8.4 *Measurement of neutrophil movement in a Boyden chamber. The furthest distance (in microns) that two or more cells have migrated into the filter is measured after a set incubation time*

Recognition or Opsonization

Recognition of foreign particles by neutrophils involves humoral factors called opsonins which act on the microorganism to render it more susceptible to ingestion by the neutrophil. The best-described opsonins (*Figure 8.5*) are antibodies of IgG class, which confer some specificity to phagocytosis, and the complement fragment C3b, generated by activation of either the classical or alternative pathways. When an opsonized microorganism comes into contact with a neutrophil, it is bound by a number of receptors: stimulation of a critical number of receptors triggers the process of phagocytosis.

Phagocytosis and degranulation

The binding of opsonized organisms to neutrophil surface receptors is followed by formation of pseudopodia which

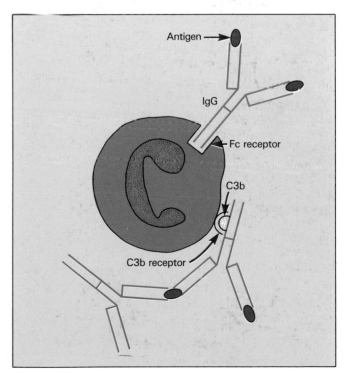

Figure 8.5 *Opsonins: binding of IgG and C3b to specific receptors on the neutrophil surface*

surround the particle. Pseudopodia formation is clearly an active process, dependent upon the formation and contraction of microfilaments.

Pseudopodia flow around the microbe, fuse and then invaginate, enclosing the organism in a vacuole called a phagosome. As the phagosome is formed, cytoplasmic granules converge and fuse with the phagosome: the granules rupture and discharge their contents. These granules are of two main types, azurophilic and specific, each containing characteristic enzymes, although lysozyme is common to both.

Bacterial killing

Phagocytosis is accompanied by a 'respiratory burst' essential to the subsequent killing of most common bacterial pathogens. The dramatic increase in oxygen consumption results from activation of an oxidase system, although the exact nature and location of this enzyme system is unclear. The oxidase reduces oxygen by one electron, generating a potent but unstable antimicrobial radical called superoxide which is further reduced by superoxide dismutase to hydrogen peroxide. Superoxide may react also with the formed hydrogen peroxide to yield reactive hydroxyl radicals. Hydrogen peroxide is a powerful oxidant and mediates oxidative microbial killing with the lysosomal enzyme, myeloperoxidase. Since hydrogen peroxide is toxic to the cell, the neutrophil apparently protects itself by metabolizing hydrogen peroxide to water and oxygen via glutathione and catalase.

All these reduced oxygen species have been detected in stimulated neutrophils, but it is not known which is the principal agent of the oxidative killing mechanism. Anaerobic conditions greatly reduce, but do not abolish, the bactericidal efficiency of neutrophils, implying that oxygen-independent killing mechanisms (*Figure 8.6*) are present also. Bacteria vary in their susceptibilies to these alternative mechanisms.

Oxygen-dependent and -independent systems together provide the neutrophil with the potential to kill and digest microbes in numbers far exceeding the requirements that normally exist.

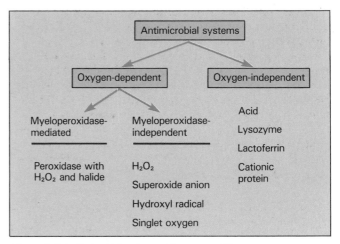

Figure 8.6 *Antimicrobial systems of the neutrophil*

The most direct and clinically useful way of identifying an abnormal predisposition to microbial infection is to show that the patient's cells are unable to kill the infecting organism as efficiently as normal cells. In standard killing assays, cells are incubated with bacteria in the presence of serum. Bacteria ingested but not killed are assayed by lysing the cells in distilled water and determining the number of residual viable organisms by culturing them on support media. Killing can also be assayed by rather simpler, if less direct, methods.

Digestion

Ingested and killed microbes obviously must be digested to prevent saturation of the neutrophils. Digestion is accomplished by the lysosomal enzymes discharged into the phagosomes. Degraded material is released from the cell into the surrounding medium.

Disordered neutrophil function

Defects in neutrophil function may be quantitative or qualitative. A critical number of circulating, functioning neutrophils clearly is required for adequate defence.

Abnormal function can be classified according to the different stages of neutrophil activity (*Figure 8.1*). Not infrequently, a number of defects may be found. However, irrespective of the basic cause, the clinical features are similar and certain generalizations are possible. Thus, infections: (1) are recurrent; (2) are prolonged; (3) respond poorly to antibiotics; (4) commonly are staphylococcal; (5) frequently involve the skin and mucous membranes; and (6) are complicated frequently by suppurative lymphadenopathy. Sometimes, recurrent infections by a restricted range of organisms give a useful clue to the possibility of a neutrophil defect (*Figure 8.7*).

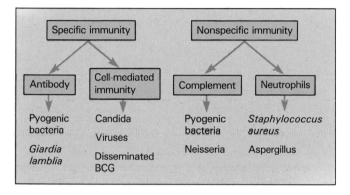

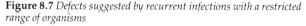

Figure 8.7 *Defects suggested by recurrent infections with a restricted range of organisms*

Neutropenia

The circulating neutrophil count usually exceeds 1.5×10^9/litre. While mild degrees of neutropenia are usually asymptomatic, moderate to severe reductions in numbers are associated with a progressive increase in the risk and severity of infection. Episodes of infection are likely to be life-threatening when the absolute neutrophil count falls below 0.5×10^9/litre.

Neutropenia may occur because of (1) abnormal stem-cell development in the bone marrow, (2) poor neutrophil release from the marrow reserve pool or (3) accelerated destruction of circulating neutrophils.

Disordered neutrophil adherence

Impairment of neutrophil adherence may be congenital or acquired.

Congenital

Patients with congenital defects of neutrophil adherence, such as the Chediak-Higashi syndrome, also have grossly abnormal neutrophil chemotaxis. The contribution made by defective neutrophil adherence to the risk of recurrent infections in these patients therefore is unclear at present.

Acquired

Drugs such as steroids, salicylates and alcohol interfere with adherence of neutrophils. Some patients with poorly controlled diabetes mellitus show abnormal adherence, the degree of impairment being related to fasting blood glucose levels, with improvement as diabetic control is established.

Disorders of neutrophil movement

Abnormal neutrophil movement may result from either an intrinsic defect of the cell itself or a failure to generate chemotactic stimuli to which the neutrophil can respond: such a failure may in turn be due either to defective release of chemotactic factors or to the presence of inhibitors or inactivators of chemotaxins.

Intrinsic cellular defects

A number of intrinsic cellular defects of polymorph chemotaxis have been described (*Figure 8.8*). While some of these can be subdivided further into abnormalities of receptor function, cellular deformability, and random or directed movement, most remain unclassified.

Persistent defects

Morphological defects Morphological abnormalities of neutrophils may impair their movement. For example, polymorphs from patients with the Chediak-Higashi syndrome show both defective chemotaxis and bacterial killing. The

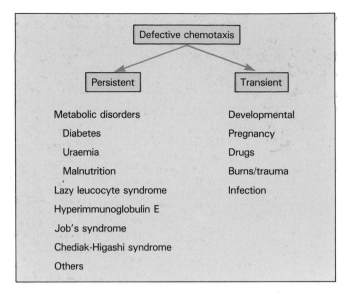

Figure 8.8 *Intrinsic cellular defects in chemotaxis*

intrinsic motility defect is due, in part at least, to abnormal cellular deformability, this mechanical restriction being partially explained by the presence of giant intracellular granules in the polymorphs.

Depressed neutrophil motility may exist without associated defects in phagocytosis or bactericidal capacity. The *lazy leucocyte syndrome* is a prototype. Affected individuals have recurrent low-grade fevers with gingivitis, stomatitis and severe neutropenia associated with poor neutrophil motility. The defect is not corrected by fresh plasma.

In some patients, defective neutrophil movement is associated with elevated serum IgE levels. The variable inheritance and phenotypic features of these patients suggest that there are multiple causes. For example, in some children, infections, severe staphylococcal abscesses, suppurative lymphadenopathy and eczema may be present, while in others there is impaired cell-mediated immunity. Patients with *Job's syndrome* have normal cellular immunity but the distinctive physical features of red hair, fair skin, dermatitis, hyperextensible joints and 'cold', nontender abscesses. Clearly, classification of this group of disorders is confused and there has been a tendency to

lump together all conditions in which there is some susceptibility to infection and a raised serum IgE. In the best characterized entity, the *hyperimmunoglobulin E syndrome*, impaired neutrophil mobility now seems to have been disproved. This is a rare disorder in which affected individuals experience severe staphylococcal furunculosis, pneumonia and repeated infections of the eyes, ears, sinuses and oral mucosa. Most have a positive family history suggestive of an autosomal dominant trait with incomplete penetrance. Characteristically, there is a markedly raised polyclonal serum IgE level, with normal levels of other immunoglobulin classes, and depressed cell-mediated immunity to specific antigens. Neutrophil mobility would seem to be remarkably normal, despite earlier reports of a chemotactic defect in this condition.

Some patients have the *immotile cilia syndrome*: this consists of abnormal respiratory tract ciliary function and poor sperm motility, in addition to a primary defect in neutrophil mobility.

Abnormal neutrophil chemotaxis has been described in association with delayed separation of the umbilical cord and recurrent, serious bacterial infections. The molecular basis for abnormal granulocyte locomotion has not yet been established. The defect is not confined to chemotaxis: abnormal bacterial killing and phagocytosis also have been found in affected infants.

Metabolic disorders   In some insulin-dependent diabetics, poor neutrophil mobility has been reversed *in vitro* by incubating the cells with glucose and insulin. While the basis of the defect is unclear, first-degree relatives of affected diabetics may show some degree of abnormal chemotaxis themselves.

Patients with chronic uraemia, severe protein-calorie malnutrition or other metabolic problems may also show an increased incidence of recurrent infection linked with impaired neutrophil mobility.

Transient defects

Various transient defects in polymorph function have been defined and may explain the increased susceptibility to infection in certain physiological and disease states (*Figure*

8.8). Neonates have impaired cell motility which improves with age and they also may fail to generate normal levels of chemotactic factor and opsonins. Pregnancy may be associated with poor chemotactic responsiveness of poly-morphs, particularly in the last trimester.

Bacterial sepsis is a major complication in patients with severe burns or surgical trauma. Impaired polymorph movement may play a role since the severity of the defect appears to correlate with the extent of injury and with decreased survival. It should be remembered that severe acute infections can affect neutrophil functions further: 'toxic' or immature polymorphs may show depressed chemotactic and bactericidal activity.

Drugs commonly impair neutrophil chemotaxis. There are many examples (*Figure 8.9*). These drugs act by breaking down the cell cytoskeleton (microtubules or microfilaments), disorganizing membrane structure, changing intracellular cyclic nucleotide levels or by other undefined mechanisms.

Deficiencies of chemotactic factors

Defective production of the chemotactic factors C3a, C5a and $\overline{C567}$ may occur in patients with primary genetic deficiencies of these components or secondary to failure of either the classical or alternative pathways of complement activation. Because neutrophils can be attracted to in-flammatory foci by other factors (*Figure 8.3*), the importance *in vivo* of these complement-derived factors is not clear. Most importantly, since activation of the complement system has a major role in opsonization of microorganisms, the heightened susceptibility to infection probably corre-lates better with defective opsonization than with deficien-cies of chemotactic factors.

Inhibitors of chemotaxis

Some disorders of defective chemotaxis have been attri-buted to the presence of inhibitory agents in the patient's sera (*Figure 8.10*). Such inhibitors may act directly on the neutrophil itself to render it incapable of reacting to chemotactic stimuli: alternatively, they may block the formation or inactivate released chemotactic factors.

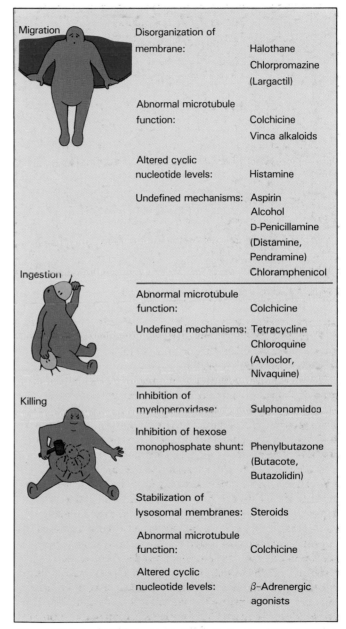

Migration		
Disorganization of membrane:		Halothane
		Chlorpromazine (Largactil)
Abnormal microtubule function:		Colchicine
		Vinca alkaloids
Altered cyclic nucleotide levels:		Histamine
Undefined mechanisms:	Aspirin	
	Alcohol	
	D-Penicillamine (Distamine, Pendramine)	
	Chloramphenicol	
Ingestion		
Abnormal microtubule function:		Colchicine
Undefined mechanisms:	Tetracycline	
	Chloroquine (Avloclor, Nivaquine)	
Killing		
Inhibition of myeloperoxidase:		Sulphonamides
Inhibition of hexose monophosphate shunt:		Phenylbutazone (Butacote, Butazolidin)
Stabilization of lysosomal membranes:		Steroids
Abnormal microtubule function:		Colchicine
Altered cyclic nucleotide levels:		β-Adrenergic agonists

Figure 8.9 *Examples of drugs or agents inducing neutrophil dysfunction*

A number of substances found in normal serum inactivate chemotactic factors: although present in low concentrations in normal serum, they occur at higher levels in certain diseases (*Figure 8.10*). Other types of inactivators, not present in normal serum, have been described in a number of conditions including active tuberculosis, alcoholic liver disease, acute leukaemia and neoplasia.

Disorders of opsonization

Severe antibody deficiency or low C3 levels from whatever cause may lead to poor opsonic function and hence to an increased susceptibility to infection. Depletion of opsonins or the presence of immune complexes may account for reported abnormalities of phagocytic function in sickle cell disease, rheumatoid arthritis and SLE.

Recently, primary defects of opsonization have been recognized. The defect can be identified by the failure of the test serum to opsonize yeast particles for phagocytosis by normal polymorphs. The abnormality is found in about 5–10% of the apparently healthy population but in over 20% of children with atopic disease or with recurrent infections of the respiratory or gastrointestinal tracts. Dysfunction of the alternative pathway of complement may be responsible. Plasma corrects the defect *in vitro* and *in vivo* and can be of therapeutic value.

Defects of phagocytosis

The best defined example of a primary defect in phagocytosis is abnormal actin polymerization. In an affected male infant with severe recurrent infections, binding of polymorphs to opsonized particles caused activation of oxidative metabolism but pseudopodia formation was impaired. Further studies showed that the amounts of actin were similar in control and patient's cells, but the patient's actin failed to polymerize normally.

Many drugs cause a secondary defect of phagocytosis (*Figure 8.9*). Colchicine is a typical example: it adversely affects microtubule function with consequent impairment of neutrophil chemotaxis and phagocytosis.

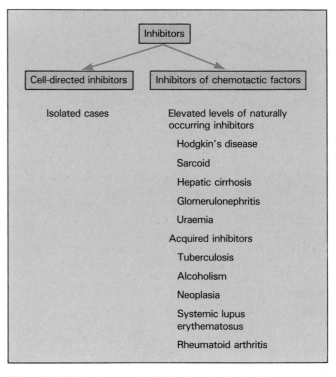

Figure 8.10 *Failure to generate effective chemotactic stimuli*

Defects of bacterial killing

When intracellular killing mechanisms fail, ingested bacteria may be able to survive and proliferate in an intracellular environment free from the effects of antibodies and most antibiotics. Several distinct syndromes are recognized.

Chronic granulomatous disease

Chronic granulomatous disease (CGD) is inherited usually as an X-linked recessive trait but an autosomal recessive form has been recognized also. It typically presents in the first month or two of life as severe skin sepsis, principally caused by *Staphylococcus aureus*, gram-negative bacilli or fungi. The most frequent complications are regional lymphadenopathy, hepatosplenomegaly, hepatic abscesses and osteomyelitis. Histology of affected organs shows multiple abscesses and noncaseating, giant-cell granulomas.

Neutrophils from patients with CGD move and phagocytose bacteria normally; however, they fail to kill infecting organisms. Infections are usually caused by catalase-producing organisms. Catalase-negative bacteria contribute to their own downfall by generating enough hydrogen peroxide to replace that which the cell fails to make. In contrast, catalase destroys the small amount of peroxide produced by the bacteria and prevents killing by CGD neutrophils.

The simplest screening test for CGD is the nitroblue tetrazolium test which depends on the ability of polymorphs to generate superoxide during phagocytosis. The diagnosis is confirmed by specific measurement of bactericidal activity. Using sensitive assays such as luminol chemiluminescence, it has become possible to diagnose the carrier state in sex-linked CGD and to make a prenatal diagnosis on fetal cells obtained at amniocentesis. It has been shown recently that males with the X-linked form of CGD lack a specific cytochrome (cytochrome b_{-245}) involved in the respiratory 'burst' needed for effective intracellular killing of bacteria. Females with CGD inherited in an autosomal recessive fashion have a normal cytochrome b_{-245} content of their cells but the machinery that reduces the cytochrome is defective.

There is no specific treatment beyond appropriate antibiotics for infections. Because most antibiotics fail to penetrate cells effectively, treatment must be continued for at least 3–4 weeks. Although the value of prophylactic antibiotics is debatable, there is some evidence that patients given continuous cloxacillin or co-trimoxazole have fewer deep abscesses. Fungal infections are important because the limited range and effectiveness of antifungal drugs makes them difficult to treat. Aspergillus is responsible usually and requires intravenous Amphotericin B for prolonged periods. In some patients, an association with a rare Kell blood phenotype (the McLeod phenotype) presents a serious potential hazard from blood transfusions.

With prompt and effective treatment, affected boys

survive longer and CGD is no longer an exclusively paediatric condition. Anecdotal evidence suggests that, in some cases, disease activity may wane after puberty.

Glucose-6-phosphate dehydrogenase deficiency

Glucose-6-phosphate dehydrogenase is essential to the hexose monophosphate shunt and hence to the 'respiratory burst'. When enzyme levels in polymorphs fall below 5% of normal, infections by catalase-positive organisms are frequent. The pattern of infection is similar to that of CGD.

Myeloperoxidase deficiency

Patients with myeloperoxidase deficiency may be asymptomatic or experience only mild infections. In contrast to CGD, the nitroblue tetrazolium test is normal but staphylococcal killing is impaired. Above normal levels of hydrogen peroxide accumulate in the phagosome and probably account for the relatively mild nature of this disorder.

Chediak-Higashi syndrome

This is an autosomal recessive disorder characterized by partial oculocutaneous albinism and the presence of giant granules in neutrophils. The failure of these granules to fuse normally with phagosomes considerably reduces the bactericidal potency of the cell, while the size of the granules interferes with neutrophil movement. Most patients suffer from recurrent skin and respiratory infections, pancytopenia, hepatosplenomegaly and progressive neurological impairment.

Treatment is confined largely to the appropriate use of antibiotics. Attempts to correct the defect using anti-metabolites, steroids or vinca alkaloids have had disappointing results. In some patients, pharmacological doses of ascorbic acid have improved in-vitro neutrophil function but the overall prognosis is usually poor.

Therapeutic considerations

Because the basic mechanisms responsible for polymorph dysfunctions are heterogeneous and mostly poorly defined, treatment for such patients is limited largely to conventional management of the complications, namely antibiotics and surgical drainage of abscesses. In recent years, some attempts have been made to correct the specific functional defects; however, responses to treatment are not uniform within the same group of patients.

In patients with complement deficiency, replacement of missing components with plasma infusions has improved chemotactic defects.

Certain drugs are known to improve leucocyte function *in vitro* and *in vivo*. Levamisole, an antihelminthic drug in cattle, possesses immunostimulatory properties and improves defective polymorph function, particularly chemotaxis, in some patients. There are anecdotal reports that *in-vitro* impairment of chemotaxis also has been corrected by preincubation of the cells with lithium chloride and that oral lithium carbonate has produced clinical improvement.

Absorbic acid also may correct defective neutrophil adherence, chemotaxis and degranulation of polymorphs. Initial reports suggested enhancement of chemotaxis and bactericidal activity in children with the Chediak-Higashi syndrome but later attempts have had mixed results.

It has been postulated that, in patients with elevated IgE levels, histamine release may be responsible for the associated depression of chemotaxis. In a few cases, competitive H_2-receptor antagonists such as cimetidine or burimamide have reversed the defect, with clinical improvement.

Conclusion

The study of patients with recurrent infections has led to the discovery of neutrophil dysfunction in a variety of diseases. In many instances, different aetiological factors may have the same result. Our knowledge of the mechanisms of normal polymorph function is incomplete, but as knowledge expands then treatment may be directed more intelligently toward specific correction of the basic defect.

Further reading

HAYWARD, A. R., LEONARD, J., WOOD, C. B. S., et al. (1979) Delayed separation of the umbilical cord, widespread infections and defective neutrophil mobility. *Lancet*, **1**, 1099–1101

JOHNSTON, R. B. (1982) Defects of neutrophil function. *New England Journal of Medicine*, **307**, 434–436

LOHR, K. M. and SNYDERMAN, R. (1981) Disorder of human leukocyte chemotaxis. *Clinical Immunology Reviews*, **1**, 67–118

SEGAL, A. W. (1980) Neutrophil function tests. *Hospital Update*, **6**, 1043–1053

SEGAL, A. W., CROSS, A. R., GARCIA, R. C., et al. (1983) Absence of cytochrome b_{-245} in chronic granulomatous disease. A multicentre European evaluation of its incidence and relevance. *New England Journal of Medicine*, **308**, 245–251

TAUBER, A. I. (1981) Current views of neutrophil dysfunction. *American Journal of Medicine*, **70**, 1237–1246

9 An overview of autoimmune disease

Introduction

We expect our immune systems to react against any foreign substance without attacking self-antigens. Until recently, immunological dogma asserted that tolerance of self-components is essential for health and hence autoimmune disease occurs only when this natural unresponsiveness to self has failed. This view presupposes that responses to self-antigens do not occur normally but it is now clear that autoimmune responses are neither abnormal nor invariably damaging. On the contrary, the ability to react against foreign antigens is related intimately to the ability to recognize self-antigens.

The fact that autoimmune responses are not, in themselves, pathogenic generates questions fundamental to our understanding of autoimmune disease: first, what mechanisms prevent the pathological expression of antiself; second, why do these mechanisms fail in some people; and third, what causes the tissue damage characteristic of the classical autoimmune diseases?

Physiological role of self-recognition

Responses to self-antigens play an essential role in initiating and in regulating immune responses. Their importance is illustrated best by the phenomenon of MHC restriction and by the idiotype network.

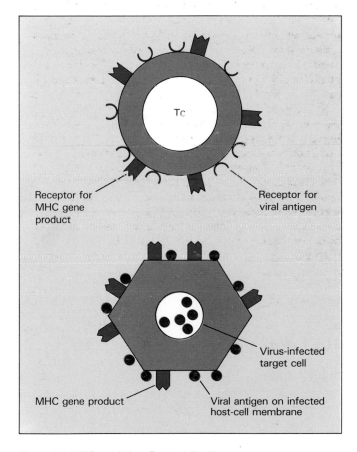

Figure 9.1 *MHC restriction. Cytotoxic T cells express one receptor that recognizes self-antigens and another that recognizes viral antigens expressed on the surface of the target cell*

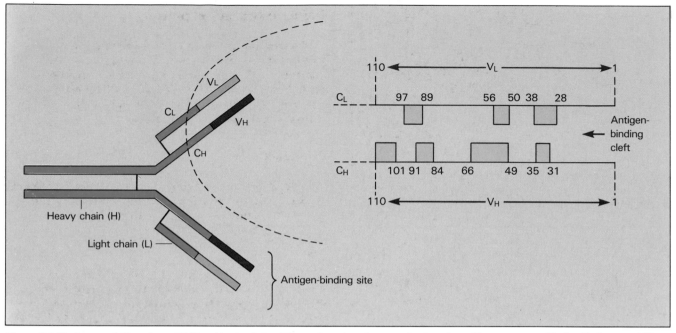

Figure 9.2 *The hypervariable regions of light and heavy chains. The numbers show the approximate amino-acid sequences constituting the hypervariable (HV) regions. Although seemingly far apart, the three-dimensional folded structure of immunoglobulins ensures that the HV regions are only about 5Å apart in the active antigen-binding site*

MHC restriction

Helper T cells cooperate with B lymphocytes and antigen-presenting macrophages in the induction of antibody responses (Chapter 6). T-cell help, however, is available only when cooperating cells are compatible at the MHC (*see Figure 7.4*). Cytotoxic T cells are essential for dealing with acute, primary viral infections but efficient killing of virus-infected, target cells occurs only if the cytotoxic T cell and the target cell are MHC-compatible (*Figure 9.1*).

This phenomenon, termed *MHC restriction*, depends upon T-cell receptors which not only recognize the foreign antigen but also the MHC antigens expressed on the stimulating cells. The nature of the T-cell antigen receptor is not certain but current evidence suggests that it is the variable region of the immunoglobulin heavy chain (V_H) (*Figure 9.2*).

Idiotype-anti-idiotype network

A comparison of the amino-acid sequences of variable regions of immunoglobulin molecules revealed three or four segments where the sequences were even more variable than elsewhere (*Figure 9.2*). These were termed the hypervariable (HV) regions. It is now recognized that the HV regions form the walls of the antigen-binding crevice of antibody molecules.

An antibody not only binds its specific antigen but is also immunogenic in its own right, *even in the animal that synthesizes this antibody*. As a result, antibodies are produced that recognize the unique antigenic determinants – the *idiotype* – contained within the HV region; the antibodies so formed are called *anti-idiotype* (*Figure 9.3*). It has been proposed that autoimmune responses to self-antigens might be regulated through a circular network of limited sets of idiotypes and anti-idiotypes.

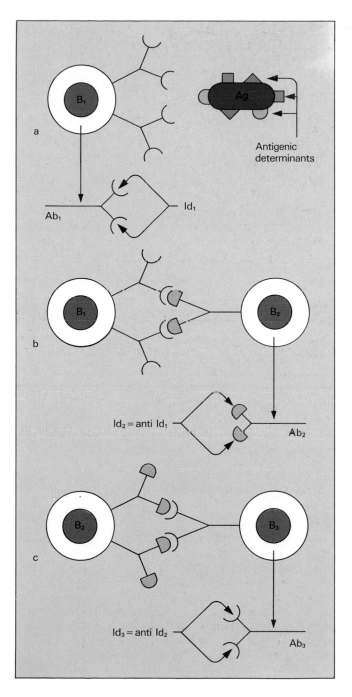

Induction of self-tolerance

If cells recognizing self-antigens are present in everyone, why does the normal immune system seem outwardly tolerant of self? A state of apparent unresponsiveness might be achieved either by 'silencing' all self-reactive lymphocytes (central tolerance) or by inhibiting the effects of these cells (peripheral tolerance).

Central tolerance

In central tolerance, no antibody is produced after antigenic challenge because the relevant B lymphocytes have been inactivated, a phenomenon termed 'clonal anergy'.

Clonal anergy

A clone is a family of lymphocytes with identical receptors for antigen. Virgin clones of lymphocytes circulate until they meet their specific antigens; then they transform and divide into many daughter cells of the same specificity. The specificity of an antibody is identical to its antigen-combining site and determined solely by structural genes beyond the influence of antigen.

It is believed that during their differentiation from stem cells into antibody-forming cells (Chapter 6), immature B lymphocytes go through a phase when contact with either self or foreign antigens induces tolerance rather than immunity. In some way, the cell receives a tolerizing signal which produces functional inactivation without cell death.

Figure 9.3 *Schematic representation of the idiotype–anti-idiotype network. In this example, the B lymphocyte clone B_1 is the dominant clone reacting to a given antigenic determinant. (a) B_1 synthesizes and secretes an antibody (Ab_1) characterized by its idiotype (Id_1). (b) Having expanded to the point where its antigen-binding receptors (and hence Id_1) reach an immunogenic level, B_1 stimulates synthesis of an anti-idiotype antibody (Ab_2 or anti-Id_1) bearing a different idiotype (Id_2) that (c) further triggers production of an anti-(anti-idiotype) antibody (Ab_3 or anti-Id_2), and so on. Animals immunized with Ab_2 (anti-Id_1) not only develop anti-(anti-idiotype) antibody (Ab_3 or anti-Id_2) but also Ab_1 (Id_1) recognizing the original antigenic determinant. Anti-idiotype clones may be either B or T cells and anti-idiotype responses can be immunosuppressive or immunostimulating*

Since B cells have a rapid turnover and are produced throughout life, this form of tolerance induction must be a continuous and active process.

Antigen blockade

Central tolerance can result also from antigen binding in circumstances which favour cell inactivation rather than cell triggering. For example, certain multivalent antigens with repeating, regularly spaced determinants can immobilize surface receptors and 'freeze' the cell membrane, while monovalent antigens may saturate the cell's antigen receptors without effecting the cross-linkage needed to activate the cell.

Peripheral tolerance

The immune system has evolved complex ways of preventing an excessive response to antigen stimulation. In peripheral tolerance, antigen-reactive lymphocytes are continually and actively inhibited by suppressor T lymphocytes, anti-idiotype antibodies or immune complexes.

Suppressor T cells may antagonize the actions of helper T cells or silence a B cell directly. Although the role of suppressor T cells in inducing tolerance and in regulating responses to conventional antigens is well recognized, the importance of these cells in inducing and maintaining tolerance to autoantigens is unproven.

Failure of immunological control mechanisms

We do not know why self-tolerance mechanisms fail in certain people. No postulated cause has achieved universal acceptance. On the contrary, studies in experimental animals suggest that autoimmune diseases result from a wide range of basic genetic and immunological abnormalities that differ from one individual to another. Disease may become apparent early in life or remain quiescent until much later, depending on whether or not exposure to 'accelerating' factors (*Figure 9.4*) has occurred.

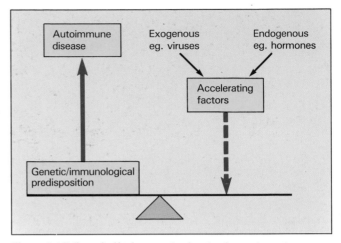

Figure 9.4 *Failure of self-tolerance. Accelerating factors determine whether autoimmune disease is expressed early or late in the life of an individual with an underlying genetic or immunological predisposition*

Immunological factors (*Figure 9.5*)

Most autoimmune diseases are characterized by the spontaneous appearance of antibodies to self-antigens. Autoantibody synthesis may result from a sudden exposure to self-antigens or from primary defects occurring at the level of the B or T cell.

Sequestered antigens

Maintenance of tolerance to foreign and self-antigens normally requires persistence of the antigen. Certain antigens, such as thyroglobulin, spermatozoa or lens proteins, were once believed to be excluded from contact with the immune system because they are sequestered in avascular sites. Any tissue damage which caused antigen release would provide an opportunity for autoantibody formation, since tolerance induction is much more difficult to achieve in adults (who possess many mature B cells) than in neonates (who have predominantly immature B cells that are readily tolerized). There is now little evidence in favour of the antigen sequestration theory for most forms of autoimmune disease. Thyroglobulin, for instance, is

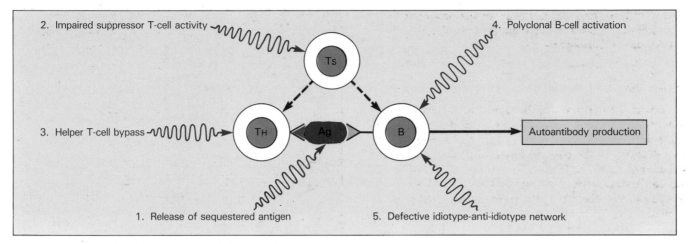

Figure 9.5 *Immunological defects that play a role in the development of autoimmune disease*

detectable in the normal circulation and perfectly healthy individuals have thyroglobulin-binding B lymphocytes in their peripheral blood. Autoantigen and self-reactive lymphocytes are clearly present in people who do not develop destructive autoimmune disease. Therefore it follows that these cells must be under some form of active restraint.

Impaired suppressor T-cell function

Many experimental and clinical studies have been interpreted as proof that autoimmune disease results from a breakdown of suppressor T-cell function. Much of this evidence has come from studies in strains of mice which develop spontaneously a disease resembling SLE: the New Zealand Black (NZB) mouse acquires autoimmune haemolytic anaemia while the offspring from mating NZB and New Zealand White (NZW) mice develop lupus nephritis. Initial reports suggested that a decline in suppressor T-cell function correlated with advancing age and parallelled the appearance of disease. It was claimed further that repeated lifelong injections of thymic cells from young mice of that strain could prevent or delay the onset of autoimmune disease. Subsequent studies, however, have failed to show any defect in suppressor cell function.

Transplantation experiments using SLE-susceptible mice and normal, but histocompatible, strains show that bone-marrow stem cells and B lymphocyte precursors can transfer the disease in the absence of T cells, strongly implying that a primary B-cell defect is responsible for SLE in this model. These and other studies cast doubt on the hypothesis that a generalized defect of suppressor T cells causes autoimmunity in animals or in man.

Helper-T-cell bypass

T and B lymphocytes differ in the ease with which they can be made tolerant of antigen. The dose of antigen needed to make peripheral T cells tolerant is over 100 times less than that needed for B cells. Furthermore, T cells remain tolerant for about 4–5 months whereas B cells return to a competent state in less than half this time (*Figure 9.6*). When exposed to small doses of antigen, B cells will either remain competent or escape from tolerance relatively quickly but T cells will become tolerant relatively easily and for a longer period. Thus, despite the presence of self-reactive B cells, self-tolerance still could be maintained by the lack of appropriate help from tolerant T cells.

Experimentally induced tolerance can be ended by immunization with cross-reacting foreign antigens or with

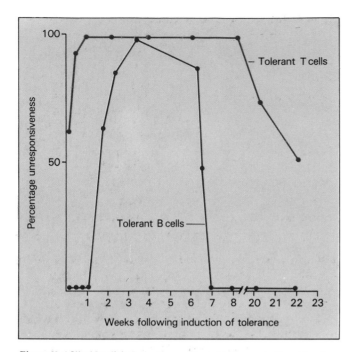

Figure 9.6 *Kinetics of the induction and loss of tolerance in T and B cells (see text for details)*

chemically altered preparations of the tolerated antigen (*Figure 9.7*). Animals made tolerant to bovine serum albumin (BSA), for instance, will lose their tolerant state after injections of chemically modified BSA or a cross-reacting antigen such as human serum albumin.

On this basis, autoimmune disease could occur if tolerant helper T cells were bypassed (*Figure 9.8*): (1) by the stimulation of different helper T cells recognizing a cross-reacting antigen; (2) by the release of nonspecific helper factors from T cells or (3) by direct stimulation of autoantigen-reactive B cells. Helper-T-cell bypass is not uncommonly seen if drugs combine directly with a self-antigen, if drugs or viruses induce expression of new antigens on the host cell surface, or if an exogenous antigen simply cross-reacts with the tolerated self-antigen.

Drug-induced autoimmune disease is well documented. A proportion of patients given α-methyldopa, for instance, develop autoimmune haemolytic anaemia. Drug-induced

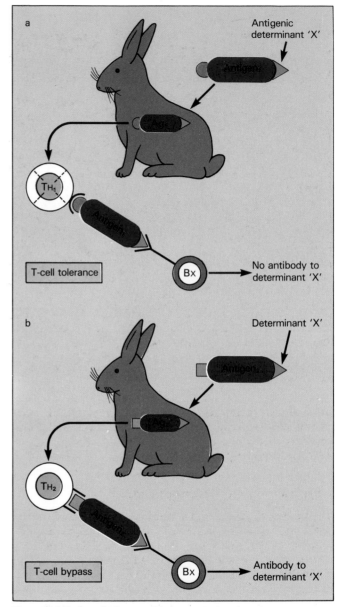

Figure 9.7 *Ending of tolerance. (a) An appropriate dose of antigen (Ag1) will induce unresponsiveness in helper T cells (TH₁) while leaving the B cell capable of reacting with small antigenic determinants ('X'). (b) A different molecule (Ag2) bearing the same antigenic determinant ('X') will provoke autoantibody production by providing a new carrier recognized as foreign by another T cell (TH₂)*

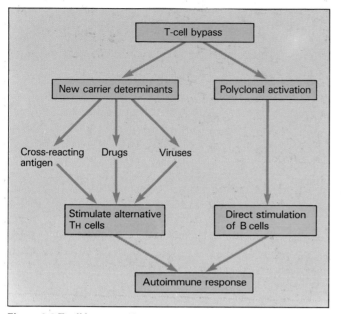

Figure 9.8 *T-cell bypass mechanisms. Unresponsive autoreactive helper T cells can be bypassed if autoantigens are linked to a new carrier to which some helper T cells are not tolerant or if autoreactive B cells are triggered by polyclonal activators*

Table 9.1 Known polyclonal B-cell activators

	Example
Viruses	Epstein-Barr virus
Bacteria/bacterial products	Lipopolysaccharide
	Staphylococcal protein A
	Lipid A-associated protein
	Mycoplasma
Parasites	Trypanosoma
	Plasmodium
Proteolytic enzymes	Trypsin
Polyanions	Dextran
Antibiotics/antifungals	Amphotericin B

lupus and production of antinuclear antibodies may follow treatment with a range of medications such as hydrallazine, procainamide or isoniazid, as well as various anticonvulsants and antibiotics.

Polyclonal activators of B lymphocytes

The primary defect of autoimmunity may lie in the B cell itself. Some clones of autoreactive B cells could possess an inherent ability to respond without needing T-cell help or, alternatively, they might be activated directly by intrinsic or extrinsic substances (termed polyclonal activators) and driven to a state of autoantibody production.

Viruses, bacteria and parasites are potent polyclonal activators (*Table 9.1*): many are associated with autoantibody production. The best known is Epstein-Barr virus (EBV). EBV produces disease by transforming B lymphocytes directly; these cells are then self-perpetuating and multiply like tumour cells. EBV infection is limited by two defences: a cellular immune response able to eliminate almost all virus-infected cells and virus-neutralizing antibodies which prevent the spread of infection from one target cell to another. The characteristic 'atypical' lymphocytes seen in infectious mononucleosis are suppressor/cytotoxic T cells seeking to limit the degree of polyclonal B cell activation and to kill infected cells.

EBV stimulation of blood lymphocytes from patients with Hashimoto's thyroiditis *in vitro* results in the appearance of detectable amounts of specific antithyroglobulin antibody of IgG class. In contrast, EBV cannot activate autoantibody synthesis in lymphocyte cultures from young, normal people but can do so in cultures from elderly individuals, a finding consistent with a decline in suppressor-cell function with age.

In general, autoantibodies induced by polyclonal activators are unlikely to be of primary relevance to naturally occurring autoimmune disease in man because: first, most polyclonal activators (with the exception of EBV) induce weakly binding autoantibodies that are mainly of IgM class, whereas tissue damage is mediated largely by IgG autoantibodies; and second, autoantibody production usually is transient and stops when the infected agent is eliminated. Nevertheless, in predisposed individuals, polyclonal B-cell activators may serve as potent accelerators of autoimmune disease.

Defects of idiotype–anti-idiotype regulation

The idiotype–anti-idiotype network plays an important role in regulating the immune system. In the case of an antibody produced to a foreign antigen, subsequent synthesis of the anti-idiotype normally suppresses the original specific humoral response. Paradoxically, however, sometimes anti-idiotype antibodies may stimulate antibody production instead (*Figure 9.3*). An antibody can therefore be viewed as the product of stimulation either by the original antigen or by an anti-idiotype antibody whose internal shape mimics that of the antigen. Specific antibodies can be induced *in the absence of antigen* by immunizing animals with anti-idiotype antibody.

Anti-idiotype antibodies can react also with cell surface receptors: the anti-idiotype structurally resembles the ligand and can mimic the action of the natural ligand on its receptor. An anti-idiotype antibody to an antibody raised against insulin, for instance, can stimulate the metabolic functions of adipocytes. Autoimmune responses could occur if anti-idiotype antibodies were to be under- or over-produced in response to antibodies recognizing self-antigens: failure to produce an anti-idiotype antibody could lead to unchecked production of autoantibodies while overproduction could also stimulate autoantibody synthesis, even in the absence of the inciting autoantigen.

The role of genetic factors

Genetic factors influence the incidence, onset and nature of many autoimmune diseases. Autoimmune diseases are linked with the genes of the MHC (*see Figure 7.4*) and with genes coding for the variable (V) and constant (C) regions of immunoglobulin molecules (*Figure 9.2*).

In Caucasians, several disorders are associated with inheritance of the HLA-DR2, DR3, DR4 or DR5 alleles (*Table 9.2*). Seropositive rheumatoid arthritis, for instance, is associated with DR4. Two distinct patterns of HLA inheritance are associated with a high prevalence of insulin-dependent diabetes mellitus. The relative risk of diabetes is increased in individuals who inherit either the HLA-B8, -DR3 or the HLA-B15, -DR4 haplotypes. This risk is increased further in those who have inherited both of

Table 9.2 Some diseases associated with inheritance of HLA antigens

HLA antigen	Disease	Relative risk*
B27	Ankylosing spondylitis	85
	Reiter's disease	37
DR2	Goodpasture's syndrome	16
	Multiple sclerosis	5
DR3	†Coeliac disease	19
	Sicca syndrome	10
	Idiopathic Addison's disease	9
	Primary biliary cirrhosis	8
	†Insulin-dependent diabetes mellitus	5
	Grave's disease	4
	Myasthenia gravis	3.5
	Hashimoto's thyroiditis	3.5
DR4	Pemphigus vulgaris	14
	†Insulin-dependent diabetes mellitus	6
	Rheumatoid arthritis	4
	IgA nephropathy	4
DR5	Pernicious anaemia	9
DR7	†Coeliac disease	5

*The relative risk is a measure of the strength of the association: it indicates how many times more frequent the disease is in individuals positive for that antigen than in people negative for it
†Some diseases show a high association with two distinct patterns of HLA inheritance

these high-risk haplotypes. In contrast, the HLA-B7, -DR2 haplotype confers some protection against developing diabetes mellitus while predisposing the individual to other disorders (*Table 9.2*). What is not clear is just how HLA genes influence susceptibility to autoimmune disease but several mechanisms have been proposed. The first, and simplest, is that of molecular mimicry. According to this hypothesis, a disease pathogen would be similar antigenically to an HLA antigen. A host which possessed that HLA type would fail to recognize the pathogen as foreign and so fail to mount an appropriate immune response. It has been suggested, for example, that *Klebsiella*, which is often found in patients with ankylosing spondylitis, shares antigenic cross-reactivity with the HLA-B27 antigen.

A second possible mechanism is that HLA antigens function as receptors for disease pathogens. Pathogens may react selectively with some but not other HLA antigens, resulting in effective induction of immunity only in individuals of a certain HLA type.

A third mechanism invokes the phenomena of Ir genes and postulates that HLA-linked Ir genes control the responsiveness to pathogenic agents. Whether or not a host develops disease after challenge with a particular pathogen would be determined then by the presence of one of these specific Ir genes. Data consistent with this model have appeared for ragweed allergy, cedar pollenosis and leprosy. It is also possible that tissue damage (perhaps caused by a viral infection) releases autoantigens which induce the Ir genes of susceptible individuals into evoking self-destructive immune responses.

The heavy (γ) chain structure of IgG varies between individuals because of the presence of allotypic determinants, called the Gm allotypes. Inheritance of certain Gm allotypes reportedly carries an increased risk of developing SLE, myasthenia gravis, insulin-dependent diabetes mellitus or Grave's disease.

The role of genetic factors has been most closely studied in strains of mice that develop spontaneous SLE-like disease: in these, genes unrelated to the MHC or immunoglobulin genes have been implicated also. The evidence suggests that murine SLE is not the result of one autoimmune gene that predisposes the individual to a wide range of autoimmune phenomena, but rather of combinations of codominant abnormal genes that are inherited independently and expressed independently. Furthermore, individual accelerating factors, characteristic for each strain, account for differences in the onset, severity and mortality of the disease. Following exposure to accelerating factors, disease is expressed early in life; in their absence, disease appears much later.

The role of hormonal factors

In general, women are far more susceptible to autoimmune disorders than men: for example, the female to male incidence of SLE is 9:1. It is likely, therefore, that chronic stimulation by sex hormones plays an important role in the expression of some autoimmune diseases.

Studies in the NZB/NZW mouse model of lupus show that androgens and oestrogens have opposing effects on the expression of disease. Disease occurs sooner in female than in male mice (*Table 9.3*). Orchidectomy accelerates the disease and giving oestrogens to castrated males accelerates it still further. Conversely, oophorectomy prolongs survival and giving androgens to castrated females prolongs it still further. In this model, oestrogens increase and androgens decrease the levels of circulating autoantibodies. A simple explanation would be that androgens enhance suppressor-T-cell function while oestrogens enhance helper T cell activity but sex hormones are also known to influence macrophage/monocyte function.

Table 9.3 Sex- and strain-differences in murine models of SLE

	50% mortality point (months)
New Zealand Black (NZB)	
Male	17
Female	16
New Zealand White (NZW)	
Male	26
Female	24
NZB × NZW hybrid	
Male	15
Female	8
BXSB	
Male	5
Female	20

The accelerating effects of female sex hormones do not apply to all forms of autoimmune disease. Ankylosing spondylitis, for instance, is far commoner in men than in women while in the BXSB model of murine SLE (*Table 9.3*), the male is also hit harder than the female. In this mouse strain, the accelerating factor is linked to the Y-chromosome and is not hormonally mediated.

The role of viruses

Virus infections could induce aberrant autoimmune responses in several ways: first, by triggering polyclonal B-cell activation; second, by selectively infecting and impairing certain subpopulations of regulatory lymphocytes, such as suppressor T cells; third, by changing autoantigens into seemingly 'foreign' proteins; and fourth, by inducing cross-reacting antibodies.

EBV, cytomegalovirus, hepatitis viruses, myxoviruses, coxsackie viruses and retroviruses are among those incriminated in autoimmune diseases in man. Most of these viruses induce autoantibodies during natural infections; some are associated also with immune complex-induced glomerulonephritis and vasculitis. However, the damaging immune complexes contain viruses and antivirus antibodies rather than self-antigens and autoantibodies. In some diseases, such as SLE, particles resembling type C RNA viruses have been seen in lymphocytes and kidneys from affected people but these particles are probably artefacts.

In contrast to human disease, evidence of a viral aetiology is established more firmly in certain animal models. Mice inoculated with Semliki Forest virus, for instance, develop a focal demyelination of their central nervous systems. An antiserum raised against cerebral gangliosides cross-reacts with virus isolated from the brains of affected mice. The virus is believed to incorporate into its envelope host glycolipids derived from oligodendrocytes. The resulting antiviral immune response causes a demyelinating state resembling multiple sclerosis in man.

Viruses and their antigenic components also play a part in the pathogenesis of murine SLE. Gp70, the major glycoprotein component of the envelope of type C RNA viruses, is found in the tissues and sera of virtually all mice. However, only SLE mice produce antibodies against Gp70 or have circulating immune complexes composed of Gp70–anti-Gp70. The presence of such complexes seems to be related to the expression of glomerulonephritis in these models.

In general, chronic viral infections are rarely the primary cause of autoimmune disease, although they do have a secondary role as exogenous accelerating factors in animals showing a genetic predisposition to develop autoimmune disease. In SLE strains of mice (*Table 9.3*), neonatal infection with lymphocytic choriomeningitis virus, for instance, shortens the 50% mortality point caused by SLE-like disease from 16 months to less than 5 months in the female NZB mouse and from 20 months to 9 months in the BXSB female.

Mechanisms of autoimmune tissue damage

The wide clinical spectrum of autoimmune diseases has been divided conveniently into 'organ-specific' and 'non-organ-specific' disease (*Table 9.4*). These conditions are considered in detail in systematic textbooks of immunology. This discussion, therefore, will deal only with the principles underlying mechanisms of tissue damage.

Table 9.4 The spectrum of autoimmune diseases

Disease	Characteristic autoantibody directed against
ORGAN-SPECIFIC	
Grave's disease	TSH receptor (thyroid-stimulating immunoglobulin)
Hashimoto's thyroiditis	Thyroglobulin; thyroid microsomes
Myasthenia gravis	Acetylcholine receptor
Insulin-dependent diabetes mellitus	Pancreatic islet cells
Insulin-resistant diabetes (associated with acanthosis nigricans)	Insulin receptor
Pernicious anaemia	Gastric parietal cells; intrinsic factor
Idiopathic Addison's disease	Adrenal cortex
Premature ovarian failure	Corpus luteum; interstitial cells
Idiopathic hypoparathyroidism	Parathyroid cells
Pemphigus vulgaris	Intercellular substance of epidermis

Table 9.4 The spectrum of autoimmune diseases (continued)

Disease	Characteristic autoantibody directed against
Bullous pemphigoid	Basement-membrane zone of dermoepidermal junction
Primary biliary cirrhosis	Mitochondria
Autoimmune haemolytic anaemia	Erythrocyte antigens (rhesus, I, etc)
Idiopathic thrombocytopenic purpura	Platelet antigens
Autoimmune neutropenia	Neutrophil antigens
Goodpasture's syndrome	Glomerular and lung basement membrane
Sjögrens syndrome	Salivary duct antigens SS-A (Ro); SS-B (La)
Rheumatoid arthritis	IgG (rheumatoid factor)
Scleroderma (CREST variant)	Centromere
Mixed connective tissue disease	Extractable nuclear antigens
Systemic lupus erythematosus	Nuclear antigens dsDNA Sm antigen IgG Lymphocytes Erythrocytes Platelets Neuronal cell antigens etc.

```
NON-ORGAN-SPECIFIC
```

Organ-specific autoimmune diseases, such as Hashimoto's thyroiditis, pernicious anaemia or Addison's disease, result from an abnormal response to a self-antigen restricted to one organ. In contrast, non-organ-specific disorders, best exemplified by SLE, are characterized by autoimmune responses to widely distributed self-antigens.

The evidence implicating an autoimmune origin for some of the listed diseases is flimsy and relatively few of the many other conditions tentatively labelled as 'autoimmune' fulfil the proposed criteria (*Table 9.5*).

Table 9.5 Criteria needed to establish an autoimmune aetiology

It should be possible to:

1. Demonstrate immunological reactivity to a self-antigen
2. Characterize or isolate the inciting autoantigen
3. Induce immunological reactivity against that same antigen by immunization of experimental animals
4. Show pathological changes (similar or identical to those found in human disease) in the appropriate organs/tissues of an actively sensitized animal

There are three main ways in which an autoimmune response causes tissue damage (*Figure 9.9*). These mechanisms are not mutually exclusive and more than one may be involved at any time.

Damage caused by autoantibodies

Autoantibodies can destroy cells or tissues, most commonly by triggering complement activation (Chapter 4) but sometimes via the actions of phagocytic or killer (K) cells, which recognize Fc receptors on IgG molecules. Examples include the autoimmune haemolytic anaemias, idiopathic thrombocytopenic purpura and autoimmune neutropenias: in these disorders, the formation of antierythrocyte, antiplatelet or antineutrophil antibodies may be primary or secondary to viral infections or drug treatment.

Goodpasture's syndrome is caused by antibodies to basement-membrane antigens found in the kidneys and lungs and characteristically, therefore, it presents as glomerulonephritis and/or lung haemorrhage. Direct immunofluorescence of an affected organ shows uniform deposition of IgG antibodies along the basement membrane, producing a smooth 'linear' pattern (*Figure 9.10*) which contrasts with the 'lumpy-bumpy' picture seen following deposition of circulating immune complexes (*see Figure 5.11*).

Many endocrine disorders are caused by autoantibodies to antigens on endocrine glands, hormones produced by these organs or the receptor sites for the hormones. About 90% of patients with insulin-dependent diabetes mellitus

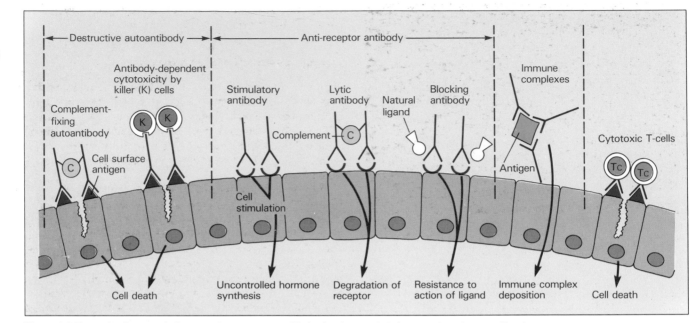

Figure 9.9 *Composite diagram of effector mechanisms responsible for the characteristic features of autoimmune disorders*

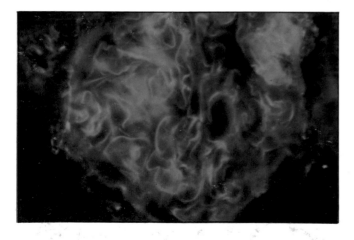

Figure 9.10 *Anti-basement-membrane antibody. A renal biopsy from a patient with Goodpasture's syndrome shows linear deposition of IgG antibody along the glomerular basement membrane*

(Type I), for instance, have islet-cell antibodies (ICA) in their sera at presentation (*Figure 9.11*); however, these antibodies are transient and fewer than 10% of this group still have ICA 5 years later. In contrast, nearly all patients with Hashimoto's thyroiditis have persistent, high-titre antibodies to thyroglobulin, thyroid microsomes and other thyroid antigens. Over one-third of patients with autoimmune thyroid disease also have circulating antibodies to gastric parietal cells while about half of those with overt pernicious anaemia have thyroid antibodies in their sera.

Autoantibodies can cause disease by stimulating or inhibiting the functions of cell surface receptors, without killing the cell (*Table 9.6*). Attachment of an autoantibody to the receptor site may have three effects (*Figure 9.9*). First, it can mimic the action of the normally activated receptor: the classic example is Grave's disease, in which a thyroid-stimulating antibody of IgG class binds to, and stimulates, the thyroid-stimulating-hormone receptor, resulting in uncontrolled production of thyroid hormones. Second, an

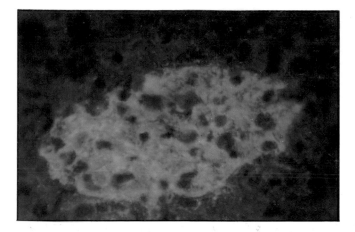

Figure 9.11 *Islet cell antibodies in a patient with insulin-dependent diabetes mellitus. The substrate is human pancreas*

Table 9.6 Anti-receptor antibodies and disease

Receptor for	Disease associated with antibody to receptor
Thyroid stimulating hormone	Thyrotoxicosis (Grave's disease)
Acetylcholine	Myasthenia gravis
Insulin	Insulin resistant diabetes
Gastrin	Pernicious anaemia
β_2-Adrenergic agonists	Asthma
Thyroid growth factor	Goitre

autoantibody may block receptor function by degrading the receptor. This occurs in myasthenia gravis, where cytotoxic autoantibodies react with the acetylcholine receptors at neuromuscular junctions. Third, the autoantibody may block the binding of the hormone to its receptor, so inducing resistance to the hormone's actions. This situation occurs in certain rare forms of insulin-resistant diabetes but more commonly in the atrophic gastritis of pernicious anaemia, where gastric parietal-cell antibodies bind to, and block, the gastrin receptors on parietal cells, inhibiting gastric acid secretion.

Damage caused by immune complexes

Immune complexes of autoantigen bound to autoantibody may be deposited in tissues throughout the body, but the kidney, joints, skin and brain are involved most frequently (Chapter 5). Activation of complement and the attraction of neutrophils and macrophages increases the inflammatory response and leads to death of bystander host cells (Chapter 4).

Immune complex deposition is responsible for many features of the non-organ-specific autoimmune diseases, such as SLE. Patients with SLE produce an array of high-titre antibodies to nuclear components (*Figure 9.12*) such as double-stranded DNA (*Figure 9.13*), ribonucleoprotein, histone, ribonucleic acid and nucleolar antigens. They also make antierythrocyte and antiplatelet antibodies that cause haemolytic anaemia and thrombocytopenia, antineuronal antibodies that may play a role in the neurological features of SLE and antilymphocytic antibodies that could interfere further with control mechanisms attempting to maintain the state of self-tolerance.

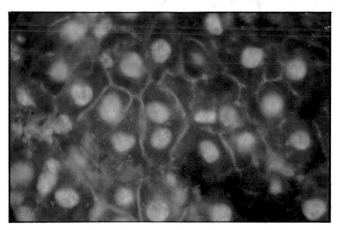

Figure 9.12 *A positive antinuclear antibody. Homogeneous staining of liver cell nuclei by serum from a patient with SLE*

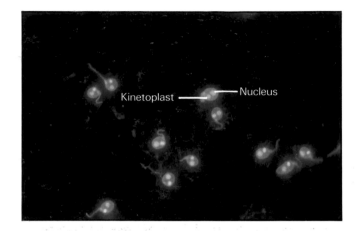

Figure 9.13 *Antibodies to double-stranded DNA.* Crithidia luciliae *is a flagellate microorganism with a kinetoplast composed of 'pure' dsDNA. Serum from a patient with active SLE stains two intracellular constituents: the nucleus and the slightly smaller, excentrically-placed kinetoplast*

Damage caused by T lymphocytes

Sensitized T lymphocytes can destroy target cells by direct cytotoxicity, by the release of lymphokines (Chapter 7) or by the recruitment of macrophages.

Although cell-mediated immunity to self antigens has been demonstrated in a wide variety of autoimmune diseases, the weight of evidence suggests that autoantibodies and/or immune complex deposition are the main routes of tissue damage.

Approaches to the management of autoimmune disorders

In view of our patchy understanding of the aetiology and pathogenesis of autoimmune diseases, it is not surprising that standard therapy has changed relatively little over the past 20 years. Current treatment is aimed largely at producing nonspecific suppression of a deranged immune system, rather than at reversing the underlying process of autoimmunity.

Less crude, and more logical, approaches to the management of autoimmune diseases in the near future can be considered under four headings (*Figure 9.14*): re-induction of self-tolerance; reversal of accelerating factors; modulation of tissue-damaging mechanisms; and replacement therapy.

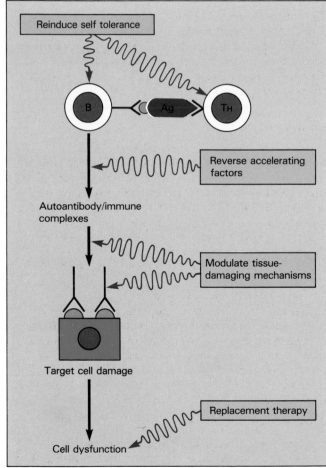

Figure 9.14 *Approaches to the management of autoimmune disease*

Re-induction of self-tolerance

Anti-idiotype antibodies

Theoretically, these could switch off synthesis of an autoantibody expressing the relevant idiotype and regulate expression of the disease. This approach has been tried with some success in animal models of autoimmune disease but may prove less successful in man because: (1) repeated injections of antisera raised in animals may cause serious immune reactions, including serum sickness (Chapter 5); (2) anti-idiotype antibodies may switch off autoantibody formation in one person yet not in another with the same disease but possessing a different idiotype; and (3) most autoantibody responses are polyclonal (Chapter 1), so an anti-idiotype antibody will only suppress one out of many clones.

Suppressor-T-cell factors

In future, these be manufactured commercially from suppressor-T-cell clones maintained in tissue culture. Crude spleen-cell supernatants, containing poorly defined suppressive factors, have been reported to prolong survival of mice with lupus-like nephritis, provided treatment was started early in the course of the illness.

Bacterial products, especially mycobacterial cell walls, are among the most powerful exogenous activators of the immune system. Synthetic copies of the immunoactive glycopeptides found in mycobacteria are called muramyl dipeptides (MDP) and have a number of biological properties. They can induce suppressor activity under certain experimental conditions. In mice, MDP conjugated to antigen can trigger T-cell-mediated suppression of the specific antibody response, but the beneficial effects of MDP linked to purified autoantigens have not yet been assessed.

Tolerance induction

Injections of purified autoantigens (e.g. nucleic acids) coupled to a tolerance-inducing carrier molecule (e.g. the animal's own IgG) have been partly successful in treating mice with SLE. The onset of lupus nephritis was delayed, especially when the injections were combined with conventional corticosteroid treatment. Immunotherapy of this type constitutes an attractive and feasible approach to SLE and other non-organ-specific autoimmune diseases in man.

In certain models of autoimmunity, such as experimental autoimmune encephalomyelitis in rats, disease can be transferred to other rats by inoculating them with autoreactive T cells which have been maintained in cell culture. Furthermore, these antigen-specific T cells can be recovered from active lesions, used to transfer the disease to other healthy recipients after a passage in culture and again isolated from areas of resulting brain damage. Attempts to induce resistance by vaccinating rats with autoreactive but attenuated clones of T cells have proved partly successful. Preliminary experiments with membrane fractions suggest that subcellular material may be as effective as living T cells in preventing experimental encephalomyelitis. Unfortunately, in many human 'auto-immune' conditions, the critical autoantigens are either unknown or in limited supply and it remains to be seen whether this exciting approach proves helpful in managing disease in man.

Bone-marrow transplantation

SLE can be prevented in genetically susceptible strains of mice by lethally irradiating them, and then transplanting bone marrow from histocompatible, normal strains; this evidence strongly implies that genetically determined abnormalities of lymphoid stem cells are primarily re-sponsible for SLE in these models. When human bone-marrow transplantation (Chapter 7) becomes a less hazardous procedure, such an approach may prove useful for severe and otherwise intractable autoimmune disease.

Reversal of accelerating factors

Drugs, viruses and hormones are the best recognized accelerating factors. Patients on drugs known to trigger autoimmune responses should be regularly screened for autoantibody formation or changed to alternative, less troublesome, medication where possible. Specific antiviral therapy is still in its infancy and, at present, has no role in the management of autoimmunity.

Oestrogens accelerate and androgens retard SLE in certain strains of mice. Regular androgen usage in humans has the serious drawback of significant and unacceptable virilization. Unfortunately, testosterone derivatives with potent anabolic but attenuated androgenic properties have been disappointing so far in treating SLE in the mouse and in humans.

Modulation of tissue-damaging mechanisms

The damaging effects of autoantibodies and/or immune complexes are largely mediated via the activation of complement and the attraction of phagocytic, inflammatory cells. Current management of many autoimmune diseases is directed towards suppressing this inflammatory response with nonsteroidal anti-inflammatory drugs, salicylates, penicillamine, gold salts and antimalarial compounds. Acute exacerbations, or more severe disease, are usually treated with high doses of corticosteroids or cytotoxic agents, such as cyclophosphamide or azathioprine. Judicious use of these drugs, coupled with increasing experience of their side effects, has improved survival considerably in many of the non-organ-specific autoimmune diseases.

Plasma exchange

Recently, plasma exchange (Chapter 5) has been used in diseases where high-titre autoantibodies (for instance, anti-basement-membrane antibodies in Goodpasture's syndrome) or circulating immune complexes (e.g. SLE) play a major role in immunopathology. On its own, plasma exchange is of limited value: its beneficial effects are transient, and a rebound of autoantibody levels can occur sometimes when treatment is stopped. Nevertheless, in severe cases plasma exchange may 'buy' enough time for conventional immunosuppressive therapy to become effective.

Total lymphoid irradiation

(Total lymphoid irradiation is a potent and unique form of therapy. Treatment consists of repeated irradiation of the lymphoid organs over a relatively short period. In murine models of SLE, TLI has reversed even well-advanced disease, with an increase in survival time, a decrease in proteinuria and a fall in anti-DNA antibody titres. Similarly, some cases of intractable rheumatoid arthritis in humans have shown a dramatic, objective decrease in disease activity which was associated with a selective reduction in the numbers and function of helper T lymphocytes. The mechanism of action of TLI is unclear: it is unlikely that radiation merely depletes those immunocompetent cells responsible for tissue damage because disease remissions outlast the recovery of cellular and humoral immunity.

Prostaglandins

Pharmacological doses of prostaglandin E_1 can increase the survival of mice with SLE. Prostaglandins have no effect on the production of anti-DNA antibodies but considerably reduce the deposition of immune complexes in the kidney and protect the animal against developing the proliferative glomerulonephritis characteristic of murine lupus.

Dietary manipulation

It is well established that protein-calorie malnutrition causes secondary impairment of host immunity. It is hardly surprising, therefore, that changes in the diet may have profound effects on animals susceptible to autoimmune disease. Low-calorie, low-fat, low zinc or restricted amino acid diets have all been shown to reduce the expression of immune complex glomerulonephritis and prolong the life span of mice with SLE-like syndromes. Such diets also reduced autoantibody production and levels of circulating immune complexes. The mechanism for these effects is unknown but the potential for treating human disease simply by modifying the diet is attractive.

Replacement therapy

Most organ-specific autoimmune disorders can be treated adequately by replacing any missing factors: thus, pernicious anaemia is best managed by injections of vitamin B_{12} and Addison's disease by cortisol and mineralocorticoids.

On the basis that autoimmunity may result from a primary defect of immunoregulatory T cells, various *thymic hormones* have been tried in mice with SLE but with very little benefit. There are few published studies of the therapeutic efficacy of thymic hormones in human autoimmune disease.

Dialysable leucocyte extracts

Extracts (Chapter 7) with specific and nonspecific effects on cell-mediated immunity have been given to patients with a variety of autoimmune disorders. The outcome of such uncontrolled clinical trials has been extremely variable so far and the efficacy of this form of treatment has been seriously questioned.

Further reading

HARRISON, L. (1982) Autoantibodies to hormone receptors. *Springer Seminars in Immunopathology*, **5**, 447–462

HOLBOROW, E. J. (ed.) (1981) Autoimmunity. *Clinics in Immunology and Allergy*, vol. 1, no. 1

KLOUDA, P. T. and BRADLEY, B. A. (1983) The interface between HLA genes and immunological diseases. In *Recent Advances in Clinical Immunology*, Number 3 (R. A. Thompson and N. B. Rose, eds). Churchill Livingstone, Edinburgh

KOFFLER, D., BIESECKER, G. and KATZ, S. B. (1982) Immunopathogenesis of systemic lupus erythematosus. *Arthritis and Rheumatism*, **25**, 858–861

MILICH, D. R. and GERSHWIN, M. E. (1980) The pathogenesis of autoimmunity in New Zealand mice. *Seminars in Arthritis and Rheumatism*, **10**, 111–147

ROSSINI, A. A. (1983) Immunotherapy for insulin-dependent diabetes? *New England Journal of Medicine*, **308**, 333–335

STRAKOSCH, C. R., WENZEL, B. E., ROW, V. V. and VOLPE, R. (1982) Immunology of autoimmune thyroid diseases. *New England Journal of Medicine*, **307**, 1499–1506

THEOFILOPOULOS, A. N. and DIXON, F. J. (1982) Autoimmune diseases. Immunopathology and etiopathogenesis. *American Journal of Pathology*, **108**, 321–365

Index

Acquired immunodeficiency syndrome (AIDS), 92–93
ADCC, *See* Antibody-dependent cell-mediated cytotoxicity
Addison's disease, 119
Adenosine deaminase deficiency, 87, 90
Adenyl cyclase, 22
Adrenalitis, autoimmune, associated with mucocutaneous candidiasis, 89
Age, and serum immunoglobulin levels, 4–5
AIDS, *See* Acquired immunodeficiency syndrome
Allergic hypersensitivity, passive transmission, 20
Allergic reactions,
  components necessary, 19
  correlation with low level of parasite infestation, 24
  genetic control, 24–25
  hereditary aspects, 24
  perennial, 28
  seasonal, 28
  variability within population, 20
  See also Atopic allergic diseases
Alopecia, associated with mucocutaneous candidiasis, 89
Alpha-chain disease, 18
Alveolitis, extrinsic allergic, 23
  immunoglobulin response, 6
Amino acid sequences, 1, 110
Amyloidosis, in myelomatosis, 11
Anaesthetic agents, intravenous, anaphylactic-like reactions, 21
Angioedema, and inherited complement defects, 43
Animals, causing allergic reactions, 28
Ankylosing spondylitis, 4
  sex related incidence, 117

Anti-idiotype antibodies, 110, 123
Antibiotics, and immunodeficiency disease, 83
Antibodies,
  deficiency: causes of, 71–76
  causes of death, 78
  complications of, 76–78
  primary, 67–71
  treatment, 81–83
  functional activity, 70–71
  natural, tests, 71
  response, in immune complex disease, 55
Antibody-dependent cell-mediated cytotoxicity (ADCC), 3
Antibody molecules, functions, 1
Antibody responses, primary and secondary, 3
Antigen–antibody reaction, 48
Antigens,
  blockade, 112
  continued exposure, and immune complex generation, 53–54
  elimination, in immune complex disease treatment, 61
  properties, 54–55
  recall, 84
  sequested, 112
Antihistamines, treatment of allergic diseases, 33
Arthus reaction, 53
Ascorbic acid, in neutrophil dysfunction therapy, 108
Asthma,
  due to house dust mite, 23
  low frequency in regions with high parasite infestation, 24
  treatment with corticosteroids, 33

Ataxia telangiectasia, and IgA deficiency, 76
Atopic allergic disease, 19
  and IgA deficiency, 76
  antigen avoidance, 32
  diagnostic tools, 28–32
  following viral respiratory infection, 27
  hyposensitization procedures, 33
  mechanisms, 19
  pathogenesis, 27
  therapies, 32–34
  See also Allergic reactions
Autoimmune disease,
  and IgA deficiency, 76
  criteria for establishing, 119
  damage caused by autoantibodies, 119–121
  damage caused by immune complexes, 121
  damage caused by T-lymphocytes, 122
  drug-induced, 114–115
  genetic factors, 116–117
  idiotype-anti-idiotype network, 110
  management, 122–125
  mechanisms of tissue damage, 118–122
  modulation, 124
  non-organ specific, 118–119
  occurrence, 109
  organ-specific, 118–119
  replacement therapy, 125
  reversal of accelerating factors, 123–124
  role of hormones, 117
  role of viruses, 118
  tolerance induction, 123
Autoimmunity,
  failure of control mechanisms, 112–118
  induction of self-tolerance, 111–112
  peripheral tolerance, 112

B-lymphocytes, 65–66
  circulating, count, 71
  in common variable immunodeficiency,
    74
  maturation pathways, 64–65
  and MHC restriction, 110
  polyclonal activators, 115
Bacteraemia, gram-negative,
  and complement activation, 41
  complement levels, 43
Bacteria, polyclonal activators of
  B-lymphocytes, 115
Bacterial infection,
  and inherited complement defects, 43
  subacute, immunoglobulin response, 6
Barriers to infection, mechanical, effects of
  breakdown, 64
Basophils,
  and allergic reactions, 19
  degranulation test, in allergic disease
    diagnosis, 31
  interaction with immune complexes, 50
Beclomethasone, in treatment of asthma,
  33
Bence-Jones myeloma, 11
Bence-Jones protein, 9
Benign monoclonal gammopathy, 14–15
Benoxaprofen, in treatment of allergic
  diseases, 33
Biliary cirrhosis, primary, immunoglobulin
  response, 6
Biopsies, to detect immune complexes, 58
Blood transfusions, 93
Blood vessels, immune complex injury, 56
Bone destruction,
  in myelomatosis, 12
  in Waldenström's macroglobulinaemia, 16
Bone marrow, in Waldenström's
  macroglobulinaemia, 16
Bone marrow infiltration, in myelomatosis,
  11
Bone marrow specimens,
  immunofluorescence, 12
Bone marrow transplantation, 93–95, 123
  complications, 95
  donor selection, 93–94
  technique, 94–95
Bronchial provocation test, 31
Brucellosis, as cause of immunodeficiency,
  80
Bruton's disease, See
  Hypogammaglobulinaemia, infantile
  sex-linked

Burimamide, in neutrophil dysfunction
  therapy, 108

Candida albicans infection, 89
Carmustine, in myelomatosis therapy, 13
carpal tunnel syndrome, in myelomatosis,
  11
Cedar pollenosis, 117
Cell-mediated immunity,
  assessment, 84
  impaired, and grafting of
    immunocompetent tissues, 93–97
  secondary causes of impairment, 92–93
  selective defects, 87–89
  therapeutic approaches to impairment,
    93–98
Cerebrospinal fluid, immunoglobulin
  levels, 7
CGD, See Granulomatous disease, chronic
CHAD, See Cold haemagglutinin disease
Chediak-Higashi syndrome, 103, 108
  defects of bacterial killing, 107
Chlorambucil, in treatment of
  Waldenström's macroglobulinaemia,
  16
Choroid plexus, immune complex injury,
  56
Chromosomal defects, and IgA deficiency,
  76
Cimetidine, in neutrophil dysfunction
  therapy, 108
Coeliac disease,
  immunoglobulin response, 6
  loss of immunoglobulins, 80
  relationship with dermatitis
    herpetiformis, 59
  with intestinal lymphoma, 7
Cold haemagglutinin disease (CHAD), 16
Complement,
  anaphylatoxins, 40
  biological effects, 39–40
  breakdown products, 41
  chemotactic activity, 40
  clinical interpretation of changes, 41–43
  collection of samples, 40
  component numbering, 35
  defects, 55–56
  definition, 35
  factor H deficiency, 44
  factor I deficiency, 44
  functional assays, 40
  immune adherence, 39
  immunochemical assays, 41

Complement (cont.)
  inherited defects, 43–46
  management, 46–47
  levels: in immune complex diseases, 42
  in infectious disease, 43
  in liver disease, 43
  in renal disease, 42–43
  low, 41
  raised, 41
  opsonization, 40
  primary C3 deficiency, 44
Complement activation, 2, 48–49
  laboratory assessment, 40–41
  modulation, 39
  pathways, 36–39
  'alternative', 36, 38
  'attack' sequence, 36, 39
  deficiencies, 45
  'classical', 36, 37–38
  defects, 44
  principles, 35–36
  results, 35
Cow's-milk-protein allergy,
  and IgA deficiency, 76
  immunoglobulin response, 7
Crohn's disease, loss of immunoglobulins,
  80
Cryoglobulinaemia, 17–18
  complement levels, 42
  treatment, 17–18
Cryoglobulins
  classification, 17
  tests, 17
Cutaneous vasculitis, and immune
  complex deposition, 58
Cylic-3', 5'-adenosine monophosphate, 22,
  23
Cyclophosphamide, myelomatosis
  therapy, 13
Cystic fibrosis, immunoglobulin response,
  6
Cytotoxic T-cells, 65

Dapsone, in treatment of dermatitis
  herpetiformis, 59
Dermatitis herpetiformis (DH),
  and immune complex deposition, 58
  relationship with coeliac disease, 59
Di George syndrome, See Thymic
  hypoplasia
Diabetes mellitus,
  associated with mucocutaneous
    candidiasis, 89

Diabetes mellitus (*cont.*)
    genetic link with autoimmune disease,
        116
    insulin-dependent, 119–120
    neutrophil motility, 104
Dietary manipulation, 124
Discoid lupus erythematosus (DLE),
    distinguishing from SLE, 58
DLE, *See* Discoid lupus erythematosus
Down's syndrome, as cause of
    immunodeficiency, 80
Doxorubicin, myelomatosis therapy, 13
Drugs, and neutrophil motility, 105
Dystrophia myotonica, 80

Empyema, immunoglobulin response, 6
Endocarditis
    immunoglobulin response, 6
    sub-acute bacterial, complement levels, 43
Endocrine disorders, 119
    associated with mucocutaneous
        candidiasis, 89
Endotoxic shock, and complement
    activation, 41
Environmental protection, 93
Enzyme replacement therapy, 98
Eosinophil chemotactic factor of
    anaphylaxis (ECF-A), preformed
    mediator, 22
Epstein-Barr virus, 115
Erythema annulare, in myelomatosis, 11

Factor VIII, paraprotein activity against, 17
Foods, causing allergic reactions, 28
    diagnosis, 32
Fungal infections, and chronic
    granulomatous disease, 107

Gamma-chain disease, 18
Gastrointestinal disease, and antibody
    deficiency, 77
Gastrointestinal infections, and IgA
    deficiency, 75
Genetic counselling, 93
Glomerulonephritis,
    and tissue deposition of immune
        complexes, 63
    complement levels, 42
    immune complex, 59
Glomerulus, immune complex injury, 56
Glucose-6-phosphate dehydrogenase
    deficiency,
    defects of bacterial killing, 107

Gluten-sensitive enteropathy,
    immunoglobulin response, 7
Goodpasture's syndrome, 119
Graft-versus-host disease (GVHD), 93, 95, 96
Granulomatous disease, chronic, 106–107
Grave's disease, 120
GVHD, *See* Graft-versus-host disease

Haematological findings, in Waldenström's
    macroglobulinaemia, 16
Haemolytic anaemia,
    and antibody deficiency, 78
    autoimmune, 89
    drug-induced, 114
    with cold haemaglutinin disease, 16
Hashimoto's thyroiditis, 119, 120
    immunoglobulin response, 6
Helminthic infestation, and high IgE levels,
    24
Helper T-cells, 65
    and MHC restriction, 110
    bypass, 113–115
Heparin, preformed mediator, 22
Hepatitis
    chronic active, immunoglobulin
        response, 6
    viral, as cause of immunodeficiency, 80
Hepatitis A, immunoglobulin response, 6
Hepatitis B, acute, complement levels, 43
Histamine,
    and allergic reactions, 19
    preformed mediator, 22
    release test, in allergic disease diagnosis,
        31
HLA-B27, 4
Hodgkin's disease, as cause of
    immunodeficiency, 80
House dust, causing allergic reactions, 28
House dust mite-induced asthma, 23
Hypercalcaemia,
    in myelomatosis, 11
    therapy, 14
Hypervariable regions, 110
Hypogammaglobulinaemia, 68
    complications, 83
    infantile sex-linked, 73
    transient in infancy, 71–73
    with IgM, 74
Hypogonadism, associated with
    mucocutaneous candidiasis, 89
Hypoparathyroidism, idiopathic,
    associated with mucocutaneous
    candidiasis, 89

Hyposensitization procedures, 33
Hypothyroidism, associated with
    mucocutaneous candidiasis, 89

Idiotype-anti-idiotype network, 110
    regulatory defects, 116
IgA,
    deficiency in atopic allergic disease, 27
    deficiency in children of atopic parents,
        27
    not detected in cord blood, 5
    selective deficiency, 69, 75–76
IgD, and disease, 8
IgE,
    age-related levels, 5, 24
    and disease, 8
    biological properties, 20
    biological role, 23–24
    discovery, 20
    hyperimmunoglobulin E syndrome, 104
    molecular structure, 20
    reaginic antibody, 19
    regulation of antibody synthesis, 24–26
        by T-lymphocytes, 25–26
    role in parasite expulsion, 23–24
    total levels, diagnostic aid, 28–29
    triggering of mediator release, 21
    unusual feature of antibody system, 23
IgG,
    correlation with age, 7
    opsonins, 101
    placental transfer, 4–5, 71–72
    selective subclass deficiency, 69, 76
IgG$_4$,
    mast cell sensitizing, 23
    reaginic antibody, 19
IgM,
    fetal production, 5
    paraproteins, 15
    selective deficiency, 69, 76
Immotile cilia syndrome, 104
Immune complex disease,
    acute serum sickness (experimental),
        51–52
    and inherited complement defects, 43
    Arthus reaction, 53
    chronic experimental, 52
    development, 44–45
    in man, 54
    treatment, 61–63
Immune complexes,
    biological effects, 48–51
    circulating, tests for, 60

Immune complexes (*cont.*)
clinical detection, 57–61
clinical implications of detection, 63
damage caused, 121
effects on lymphocyte function, 51
failure to eliminate, 54
inflammatory responses to deposition, 49
interaction with cells, 50
limitations of assays, 60–61
normal clearance, 53
pathological effects of deposition, 56–57
persistent generation, 53–56
removal, in treatment, 62
Immune response, manipulation, in
treatment of immune complex disease,
62
Immune response genes, 4
Immune system,
nonspecific immune mechanisms, 66
specific mechanisms, 64
Immunization,
and impairment of cell-mediated
immunity, 93
ending experimentally induced
tolerance, 113–114
tests, 71
Immunodeficiency,
cellular basis, 64–66
classification, 66–67
common variable, 74
laboratory tests, 70–71
severe combined (SCID), 89–90
with thymoma, 74–75
Immunoglobulin,
intramuscular, reactions to, 81–82
levels, immunodeficiency tests, 70
replacement therapy, 81
secondary causes of deficiency, 79–80
Immunoglobulins,
abnormalities, 5–8
age-related serum levels, 4–5
basic structure, 1
binding to cells, 2–3
classes, 1–2
increased loss, 80
monoclonal, *See* Paraproteins
patterns in disease, 6
placental transfer, 3, 4–5
significance of raised serum levels, 6
structure versus function, 2–3
Immunosuppressive drugs, as cause of
immunodeficiency, 80

Infections,
and antibody deficiency, 76–77
as cause of cell-mediated immunity
impairment, 92
as cause of immunoglobulin deficiency,
80
complement levels, 43
complicating bone marrow
transplantation, 95
environmental protection from, 93
immunoglobulin response, 6–7
neutrophil motility, 105
Inflammatory bowel disease,
immunoglobulin response, 7
Inflammatory response, 49
Intestinal infection, immunoglobulin
response, 6
Intestinal lymphangiectasia, loss of
immunoglobulins, 80

'Lazy leucocyte syndrome', 104
Lens proteins, 112
Leprosy, 117
and immune complex deposition, 58
as cause of immunodeficiency, 80
immunoglobulin response, 6
Leucocytes, dialysable extracts, 125
Leukaemia,
acute, as cause of immunodeficiency, 80
and immunodeficiency, 98
chronic lymphatic, 16, 79
Leukotrienes, newly formed mediators, 22
Levamisole, neutrophil dysfunction
therapy, 108
Lipoproteins, paraprotein activity against,
17
Lithium carbonate, in neutrophil
dysfunction therapy, 108
Liver, fetal grafts, 96
Liver disease,
and antibody deficiency, 77
complement levels, 43
immunoglobulin response, 7
Lymphocytes,
immune complex effects on function, 51
total count, 85
transformation, 85–86
Lymphokine, release, 86
Lymphomas,
intestinal complicating coeliac disease, 7
malignant, 16

Lysis,
as result of complement activation, 35
of invading microorganisms, 49
Lysosomal enzymes, in parasite expulsion,
23
Lysosomal enzymes, preformed mediator,
22

'M' components, *See* Paraproteins
Major histocompatibility complex (MHC), 4
genetic link with autoimmune disease,
116
restriction, 109, 110
Malaria,
complement levels, 43
as cause of immunodeficiency, 80
Malignancy,
and immunodeficiency, 78, 79
related to paraproteins, 9
Malnutrition, as cause of cell-mediated
immunity impairment, 92
See also Protein-calorie malnutrition
Mast cells,
and allergic reactions, 19
degranulation, 3, 23
interaction with immune complexes, 50
sensitizing antibodies, 23
stabilization, 33
Measles, as cause of immunodeficiency, 80
Mediators,
effects, 22–23
modulation, in treatment of immune
complex disease, 62–63
newly generated, 22
pharmacological neuralization of effects,
33
preformed, 22
species difference in relative importance,
22–23
triggering, 21
Melphelan, in myelomatosis therapy, 13
MHC, *See* Major histocompatibility
complex (MHC)
Monoclonal immunoglobulins, *See*
Paraproteins
Monoclonality, 5–6
Mononucleosis, infections,
as cause of immunodeficiency, 80
immunoglobulin response, 6
Moulds, causing allergic reactions, 28
Mu-chain disease, 18
Mucocutaneous candidiasis, 89, 98

Multiple sclerosis, IgG levels in
  cerebrospinal fluid, 7–8
Myeloma,
  Bence-Jones, 11
  biclonal, 11
  multiple, as cause of immunoglobulin
    deficiency, 80
  staging by cell mass, 12
Myelomatosis, 10–14
  clinical features, 11
  diagnosis, 10
  incidence, 10–11
  investigations, 11–12
  management of complications, 14
  myeloma staging by cell mass, 12
  neoplastic plasma cells, 11–12
  paraprotein types, 11
  prognostic factors, 13
  therapy, 13–14
Myeloperoxidase deficiency, defects of
  bacterial killing, 107

Nasal provocation tests, 31–32
Neisseria infections, and inherited
  complement defects, 43
Nephritis, complement levels, 43
Nephrotic syndrome, 80
Nervous tissue, paraprotein activity
  against, 17
Neutropenia, 103
  autoimmune, and antibody deficiency,
    78
Neutrophil chemotactic factor (NCF),
  preformed mediator, 22
Neutrophils,
  adhesion, 99
    disordered, 103
  bacterial killing, 102
    defects, 106–107
  chemotaxis: deficiencies, 105
    inhibitors, 105–106
  circulation, 99
  degranulation, 101–102
  development, 99
  digestion, 102
  dysfunction, 102–103
    immunoglobulin response, 6
    therapies, 107–108
  interaction with immune complexes, 50
  major role, 99
  movement, 99–100
    disordered, 103–105
  normal function, 99–102

Neutrophils (cont.)
  opsonization, 101
  disorders, 106
  phagocytosis, 101–102, 102
    defects, 106
Non-Hodgkin's lymphoma, as cause of
  immunodeficiency, 80

Osteomyelitis, immunoglobulin response,
  6
Osteoporosis, in myelomatosis, 12

P–K reaction, 20
Panhypogammaglobulinaemia, 67
Papain, action on immunoglobulins, 1
Paraproteinaemia, distinguishing benign
  from malignant, 14
Paraproteins,
  age-related levels, 9
  clinical significance, 9
  IgM, 15
  types in myelomatosis, 11
  with antibody activity, 16–17
  See also Benign monoclonal gammopathy
Parasite infestation, role of IgE in
  expulsion, 23–24
Parasites, polyclonal activators of B
  lymphocytes, 115
Pernicious anaemia, 119
  associated with mucocutaneous
    candidiasis, 89
Phagocytes,
  dysfunction, 56
  mononuclear, interaction with immune
    complexes, 50
  receptors, 2
Placental transfer, 3, 4–5
  of IgG, 71–72
Plasma cells, neoplastic, in myelomatosis,
  11–12
Plasma exchange, autoimmune disease
  therapy, 124
Plasma infusions, immunoglobulin
  replacement, 82
Plasma volume expanders, anaphylactic-
  like reactions, 21
Plasmapheresis,
  treatment of cryoglobulinaemia, 18
  treatment of Waldenström's
    macroglubulinaemia, 16
Platelet activating factor (PAF), newly
  formed mediators, 22

Platelets, interaction with immune
  complexes, 50
Pollens, causing allergic reactions, 28,
  117
Polyclonal hyperimmunoglobulinaemia,
  6–8
Polyclonality, 5–6
Portal cirrhosis, immunoglobulin
  response, 6
Prenatal diagnosis, 93
Prostaglandins,
  autoimmune disease therapy, 124
  newly formed mediators, 22
Protein-calorie malnutrition,
  as cause of immunodeficiency, 79
  neutrophil motility, 104
Protein-losing enteropathy, 80
Provocation tests, in allergic disease
  diagnosis, 31–32
Pruritis, in myelomatosis, 11
Purine nucleoside phosphorylase
  deficiency, 87, 88–89
Pyoderma gangrenosum, in myelomatosis,
  11

Radio allergosorbent tests (RAST), 29–30
Radiocontrast media, anaphylactic-like
  reactions, 21
Ragweed allergy, 117
RAST, See Radio allergosorbent tests
Raynaud's phenomen, 16
Reagins, 19, 20
Recall antigens, 84
Renal biopsies, immune complex disease,
  59
Renal disease, complement levels, 42
Renal impairment, in myelomatosis, 11
Respiratory infection,
  acute, immunoglobulin response, 6
  and antibody deficiency, 76–77
  and IgA deficiency, 75
  viral, atopic allergic disease following,
    27
Rheumatic disease,
  and antibody deficiency, 77–78
  complement levels, 42
  genetic link with autoimmune disease,
    116
  immunoglobulin response, 7
Rheumatoid factor, 17
Rubella, as cause of immunodeficiency, 80

132

Schistosoma mansoni, immunity against, 23
SCID, *See* Severe combined
    immunodeficiency
Severe combined immunodeficiency
    (SCID), 89–90
    associated with adenosine deaminase
        deficiency, 90
    with immunoglobulins, 90–91
Skin,
    active sensitization, 84
    delayed hypersenitivity reactions, 84
    immune complex injury, 56
Skin biopsies, to detect immune
    complexes, 58
Skin tests, in allergic disease diagnosis,
    30–31
Skull, osteolytic lesions, in myelomatosis,
    12
Sodium cromoglycate, 33
Spermatozoa, sequestered antigens, 112
Spinal cord compression,
    in myelomatosis, 11, 12
    therapy, 14
Subacute bacterial endocarditis,
    immunoglobulin response, 6
Subphrenic abscess, immunoglobulin
    response, 6
Suppressor T-cells, 65, 123
    impaired function, 113
Synovium, immune complex injury, 56
Syphilis, as cause of immunodeficiency, 80
Systemic lupus erythematosus (SLE), 119
    cerebrospinal fluid estimation, 7
    complement levels, 42

Systemic lupus erythematosus (SLE) (*cont.*)
    distinguishing from DLE, 58
    immunoglobulin response, 6
    sex-related incidence, 117
    and tissue deposition of imune
        complexes, 63

T-lymphocytes,
    count, 85,
    damage caused by, 122
    in common variable immunodeficiency,
        74
    maturation pathways, 64–65, 65
    subsets, 85
    See also Helper T-cells; Suppressor T-cells
Thrombocytopenia, autoimmune, and
    antibody deficiency, 78
Thromboxanes, newly formed mediators,
    22
Thymic factor, 97
Thymic hypoplasia, 88
Thyoma, associated with
    immunodeficiency, 74–75
Thymus, fetal grafts, 97
Thyroglobulin, sequested antigens, 112
Tissues,
    factors affecting immune complex
        deposition, 56
    mechanisms of immune complex injury,
        56–57
Total lymphoid irradiation, autoimmune
    disease therapy, 124
Tourtellotte's formula, 7
Transfer factor, 92, 97–98

Trypanosomiasis, as cause of
    immunodeficiency, 80
Tuberculosis,
    as cause of immunodeficiency, 80
    immunologlobulin response, 6

Ulcerative colitis, loss of immunoglobulins,
    80
Uraemia, neutrophil motility, 104

Vaccines, response variability, 4
Vasoactive amines, release, 3
Vasomotor reactions, to intramuscular
    immunoglobulin, 81–82
Viruses,
    polyclonal activators of B-lymphocytes,
        115
    role in autoimmune disease, 118
Vitiligo, associated with mucocutaneous
    candidiasis, 89

Waldenström's macroglobulinaemia, 15–16
    clinical features, 15–16
    investigations, 16
    prognosis, 16
    symptoms, 15
    treatment, 16
Wiskott-Aldrich syndrome, 91–92, 98

Xanthomata, in myelomatosis, 11

Yeasts, causing allergic reactions, 28